Practical guides to homeopathy

A practical guide to

methods of homeopathic prescribing

Ellen Kramer MCPH
Director, College of Practical Homeopathy (UK)

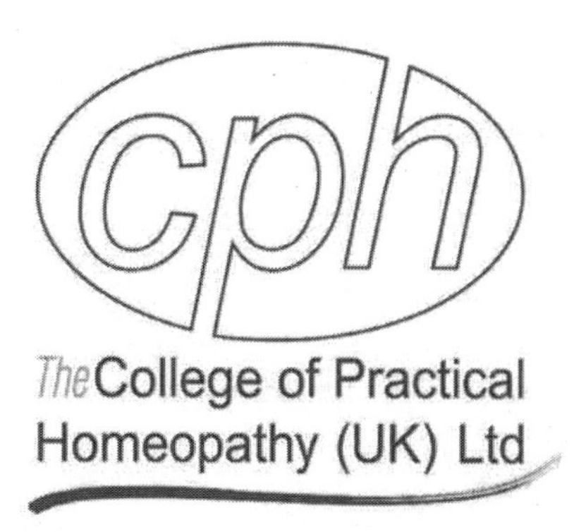

A practical guide to methods of homeopathic prescribing
by Ellen Kramer MCPH

ISBN 978-0-9555552-0-6

Published by Farkram Ltd in conjunction with
The College of Practical Homeopathy

WRITERSWORLD, 9 Manor Close, Enstone, Oxfordshire OX7 4LU, UK
Website:www.writersworld.co.uk

THE COLLEGE OF PRACTICAL HOMEOPATHY
760 High Road, North Finchley, London N12 9QH, UK.

Tel: (44) 020 8445 6123
E-mail: admin@collegeofpracticalhomeopathy.com
Website:www.collegeofpracticalhomeopathy.com

Registered in England and Wales: Number 4781658:
Registered Office: 111 Charterhouse Street, London EC1M 6AW

Printed and bound by CPI Antony Rowe, Eastbourne
Illustration and design by Geraldine Alferoff. Tel: 01547 528370.

The author

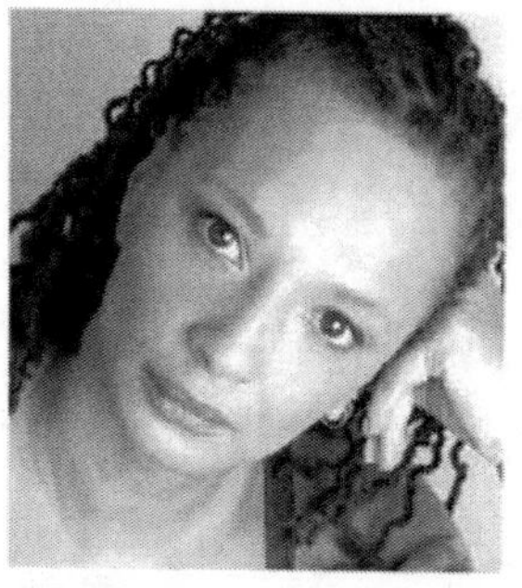

Ellen Kramer LCPH, MARH
is Director and Course Manager for the **College of Practical Homeopathy (UK) Ltd**, who provide the only full-time and part-time 'practical' training courses in London. She also has busy private practices in Islington and Finchley.

'Having spent several years running a large complementary health centre with a range of practitioners, and having co-founded a training college I began to notice a real difference between the successful practitioners and those that found it difficult to sustain a practice. It was clear to me that a good training in a complementary medicine was not enough to ensure success as a practitioner – a change in mental attitude is also required. Homeopathy needs to be seen as a reputable, accountable and independent health profession, and we need to improve standards of training and education across the sector to help achieve this.

I want to be part of a profession that has enough knowledge, expertise and confidence to present a strong and credible alternative approach to dealing with sickness and disease in our society. One that is willing to face the challenges that homeopathy will face in the twenty-first century from an array of vested interests in keeping control over peoples health.'

Practical guides to homeopathy

This is the first in a series of *Practical guides to homeopathy*.
If you are interested in finding out when the next guide is being published please check our website (shown on the previous page).

Dedication

This book is dedicated to all the great homeopaths and healers who walked before me and dared to keep the art of healing simple. Clinical prescribers such as Dorothy Shepard, Ellis Barker, Dr John Clark, Dr Compton Burnett and Robin Murphy have all inspired me to keep searching for the answers like a true detective. I would also like to make a special dedication to Robert Davidson, who in my darkest moments of despair reminded me of my true calling, challenged me to try again and inspired me to bring together a clear treatise on methods as a practical tool for practitioners and students in the science and art of healing.

Contents

With thanks to

Caroline Gaskin for her invaluable contribution to the material in this book and to making methodologies easy to apply.

The many patients and students who have kept me developing and evolving (and no doubt will continue to do so!) as a practitioner, teacher and healer.

Tim Lloyd and all the tutors at **The College of Practical Homeopathy (UK)** who believed in me and have supported the college's unique approach to producing homeopaths fit for the twenty-first century.

Poppy Altmann, Anne Campbell, Mandy Redman, Sandy Pepper, Adriana T. Candeias and Geraldine Ford for their comments on various drafts and Geraldine Alferoff for her support and patience in getting the material ready for publishing.

Tony Farley, who is the only one who really knows what it took to get here – without him this would not have been possible.

Foreword

Homeopathy is the science of individuality. The science of measurement and statistics has a long way to go before it is mature enough to be able to deal with the individual event. The astonishing elegance of Hahnemann's *Principle of Similars* is probably one of the great developments in human thinking, similar to the invention of the idea of zero.

A principle has no fixed method of application. This means that there are an unknown number of ways of applying the *Principle of Similars*.

This book is a very competent exploration of some of the better tested methods in clinical use. Explore them with an open mind for they all work with the patients they are best suited for. No method will work on every patient. None. The trick, as they say, is to find the similarity and that is defined by the overarching therapeutic question 'what is to be cured, right now?' This question is what defines therapies and the varying methodologies of those therapies.

Each of us needs to be taught the necessary clinical and observational flexibility to be able to answer that simple question for each of our individual patients. Otherwise, as the old saying goes 'if you only have a hammer, then everything has to be a nail'.

This book of proven methods is a fine way to expand your tool-kit far beyond the classical 'hammer'. I would advise you to read it many times, using it as a base for a process of wonderful expansive ongoing learning. Used with courage and persistence these methods and their individual application will greatly increase your value to your patients and increase your own satisfaction in your mission of cure.

Robert Davidson
FSoH, FHMA, MCPH, MCOH, MARH

Introduction

It has become increasingly obvious as I have taught students, run seminars and trained tutors over the past decade that there is a real gap in the understanding of the range and use of the different methods available to support homeopaths.

The 'classical' method is often seen as synonymous with homeopathy, but is only one of a number of different methods available for practitioners to use. Many students and practitioners are trained to use only this one method. Although this can be successful in some cases, it is fraught with all kinds of problems for the prescriber and the patient (for example the 'aggravation' and the 'healing crisis').

All disciplines grow and develop on those that preceded them. Homeopathy is no exception to this. In the early days of homeopathy, prescribing was done on just a few chosen symptoms. This process is still used successfully in cultures whose natural body defences have not been interfered with in a major way (by the introduction of modern drugs, immunisation programmes and changes in the natural diet).

By the beginning of the twentieth century dealing with human health was becoming more complex. People were being exposed to diseases outside the normal disease state for their culture. This was further complicated by the suppression of symptoms by drugs and vaccinations.

By the end of the twentieth century humanity had reached what has been described as the **degenerative** period, particularly in Westernised societies where nutritionally deficient diets, stress, pollution and an over-emphasis on an allopathic approach to illness predominated.

It is increasingly clear to us that the twenty-first century will be the **collapse** period. Large numbers of the population are beginning to suffer from partial or total immune system breakdown (AIDS, allergies, ME, all kinds of cancers) As well as parasites and viruses, we are now exposed to chemicals ranging from pesticides and insecticides in our food to toxins in everything from hair dyes to cosmetics, paints and solvents. A recent report by Greenpeace and the World Wide Fund for Nature found that newborn babies are being contaminated with a toxic cocktail of dangerous chemicals. The concern is that this toxic cocktail can affect our mental and sexual development, and is linked to birth defects, chronic disease, cancers, allergies, and learning and behavioural difficulties.

The importance of this for those joining the profession and for working homeopaths is that dealing with the effects of this level of toxicity is now a major part of practice. Successful practitioners need strategies for dealing with this. Methods for prescribing are no longer as clear cut.

The complex pictures presented by the modern patient need to be matched by an understanding of the variety of methods available, and which particular method is the most appropriate at particular points along the healing process. An understanding of the main methods developed so far, and their strengths and drawbacks, is a fundamental part of the development of the homeopath.

With all methods the formulation of an accurate and detailed time-line is invaluable. A time-line helps to organise the patient's case into a manageable format. This helps to clarify cause, effect and need for cure.

All methods produce a prescription which is styled individually according to the chosen method.

By understanding the different methods we can ensure that homeopathy continues to grow, develop and evolve to meet the ever increasing levels of suppression and toxicity that our modern twenty-first century patients will present.

I hope you will find this book instrumental in advancing your professional understanding of the different methods, and that it will give you a deeper insight into the philosophy and practice of homeopathy. Methods are not rules but guides, acting as a structured foundation, freeing the prescriber to become more creative. You can only become a successful practitioner when you know how to apply them and understand their limitations.

Ellen Kramer MCPH, Director
The College of Practical Homeopathy (UK)

A beginning is the time for taking care that the balances are correct. To begin your study of homeopathy then, take care that you place the guidance of your study in the hands of those that have a genuine interest in both the subject and in you, and that they can demonstrate an enthusiasm for life and growth. Look beyond the superficial and the sound bites and seek a deeper perspective of those that you would have as your teachers.

Tony Farley M.Phil (Cam)

Chapter 1

The basic tools of homeopathy

A successful homeopath needs to understand the underlying principles of homeopathy and be able to use appropriate methods and practical applications to produce the required result – restoring health to the sick.

Samuel Hahnemann believed that approaches to disease must be studied from the viewpoint of vitality (the life and health of an individual) and not from the study of disease and the suppression of symptoms. He believed that we have a vital energy that will keep the body not only alive but healthy, unless it is disturbed in some way. These disturbances show themselves as physical, emotional or mental problems.

Symptoms are manifestations of the 'vital energy' seeking to restore its natural balance and may be used as indicators of how treatment should proceed. Disease is unique to each individual depending on their particular susceptibility.

Homeopathic treatment is based on the concept that 'like cures like' (the principle of similars) in that what can cause symptoms can also cure them (the simillimum).

Homeopathic remedies can be sourced from the mineral, vegetable, animal and human kingdoms. Their value to the 'simillimum' is determined by traditional herbal usage, poisoning, clinical experience and 'provings' (tests on healthy people).

A crucial aspect of homeopathy is that prescriptions should be based on the minimum dosage necessary to activate a return of the vital energy to a balanced state. To achieve this Hahnemann developed the practice of 'serial dilution' (now called potentisation) by which substances were reduced to micro dosages by dilution and impact.

It is important to understand that homeopathy comes from a fundamentally different philosophical perspective to allopathy (modern western medicine). Remedies do not operate in the same way as modern drugs – although some homeopaths seem to prescribe from that perspective!

Samuel Hahnemann believed we should aim to support the natural vital energy in its work of keeping us healthy.

These basic principles are taken from his 6th Organon and underlie the science and art of homeopathy:

1. The homeopath's mission is to restore health to the sick. We call this healing.
2. Healing should be accomplished in the most speedy, gentle and reliable manner.
3. The homeopath should try to be an unprejudiced observer so they can see the patient's real state of health and be able to recognise relevant and perceptible signs of disease.
4. Every homeopath, in their role as healer, must have a good understanding of what causes and sustains illness and how to help the patient heal themselves.
5. To support the patient in this process of healing, the homeopath must discover the underlying cause while respecting the individuality of the patient's constitution (mental, emotions, physicals etc).
6. To do this, the healer must get to know the state of the patient and be able to select the correct remedy, dose and repetition according to each individual case.
7. In every individual case you must look at the totality of the symptoms within the context of the cause or causes of the disease.

It follows therefore that homeopathy is both an art and a science.

The science of homeopathy is in the:

- careful analysis and evaluation of the vital energy of the patient
- evidence of what needs to be cured
- choice of the most appropriate method and its application.

The art is in:

- understanding the best use of the repertory
- choosing remedies, the potency and how the prescription is given.

This should culminate in the stimulation of the vital energy with a successful result for the patient.

If you put these basic principles into practice, returning to them when confused, they will act as an anchor to keep you linked to the underlying philosophy of homeopathy.

Homeopathic principles and a wider context

As a homeopath you need not only a good grounding in the basic principles of homeopathy but also a knowledge and understanding of the wider history and philosophy of healing through the ages. This will help you to put a homeopathic approach in context.

To become a homeopath who can deal with the myriad complaints that patients will present you with, you will need:

1. A clear understanding of anatomy, physiology and pathology *(principles 3 and 4)*

- Anatomy is the study of the physical body.
- Physiology is the study of how all the different parts work (or don't work) together.
- Pathology is the study of how it goes wrong.

Your patients will normally start by telling you about their pathology – what they think is wrong with them and the symptoms they are worried about. As a professional homeopath, your business is to develop a deeper understanding of the underlying disease from the symptoms they tell you, and be able to relate this to your knowledge of how things should work in a healthy person. This will help you to understand the cause of their symptoms, not just from an allopathic perspective but more importantly from a homeopathic perspective.

To be able to place these symptoms into a context you will need to understand why the body is presenting these symptoms. An understanding of how the physical body operates will help you do this. It will also help you to understand any medical terminology used by the patient and be able to explain what is going on for them in everyday language.

By keeping level-headed (when all about you are losing theirs as they focus on the symptoms) you can choose a treatment strategy that supports key organs and is tailor-made for your patient.

Another important tool is an up-to-date book on drug side-effects. The clinical trials on drugs can be viewed as basic provings, the recognised side-effects will tell you how those drugs poison people and the key organs affected – you can use this information to help you adjust your treatment strategy.

The knowledge-base developed by allopaths and the diagnostic tools available to them are very useful tools to have at your fingertips. They will help you understand what is going on for your patient. Allopathy has provided a clear map of the human body, alongside many useful diagnostic tools, so why not use them to support your treatment strategy?

2. Knowledge of other energy paradigms *(principles 3 and 4)*
Three main energy models have developed in different cultures. These provide useful insights for homeopaths. Their common theme is that they are all based on 'observation by astute healers' over many centuries (an unrivalled grounding in empirical science). Each of these has a complete body of knowledge, with its own paradigms and parameters. They are:
- the meridian system
- the chakra system
- the human energy or auric field.

Common key issues to remember
- The terms 'life force', 'vital energy', 'qi', 'chi' etc are not 'new age' concepts but have a very long history in patient care and medical theories.
- This history has been suppressed to a great extent by the rise of 'allopathic', so called 'scientific', medicine in the last two centuries.

Homeopathy takes an essentially eclectic approach to health
- it works on an energetic level by supporting the 'vital energy'
- it follows a philosophy of minimal intervention
- it can be combined in a holistic approach with nutrition, herbal treatment and other non-invasive therapies.

3. Good powers of observation *(principle 3)*
Homeopaths must become good observers and astute evaluators of all that is going on with their patients. A wider understanding of healing paradigms and a good basic knowledge of anatomy, physiology and pathology from a homeopathic perspective will help you to make links between the mind and body, and to view symptoms presented in a deeper and wider context. This will help you to avoid becoming a remedy chaser, using increasingly more esoteric methods of guessing the remedy, or beginning to see or use remedies as alternative allopathic drugs.

The more you can begin to 'see' the physical and emotional state, the presenting (and hidden) symptoms and their possible causes, and relate them to basic principles, the better you become at finding and treating the obstacles to cure. Developing your powers of observation helps you to ask the right questions. This is the real art of homeopathy!
Bear in mind: cause – effects – and obstacles to cure.

Essential tool-kit for the homeopath

1. Ability to take a case and a time-line *(principles 5, 6 and 7)*
This will help you to place the symptoms your patient tells you into a context. Everyone reacts differently to the trials of life and as a consequence will present different symptoms of stress with varying levels of severity. It is the ability to deal with this 'individuality' which is one of the strengths of homeopathy.

Through clinical experience and observation, homeopaths have noticed that if the true cause of disease is not addressed, the vital energy becomes weaker with each successive generation. From a homeopathic perspective this is caused by the suppression of symptoms by:

- the increase in vaccinations
- the abuse of steroids
- the use of synthetic oestrogens
- the drastic rise in the use of increasingly sophisticated and toxic drugs.

Natural childhood illnesses play a vital role in maturing the immune system, but if they are suppressed by vaccination and drugs they can be a shock to the vital energy. This is especially true in those who are nutritionally deficient or immune-compromised.

The alarming increase in surgical interventions (which are also a shock to the vital energy) can also lead to long-term chronic illness with serious consequences for the vital energy of the individual.

It is important to use a time-line to record the sequence of events that lead to the presenting symptoms. It is a useful shortcut to help you see root causes of diseases *(principle 2 – in a speedy, gentle and reliable manner).*
Having now gained an appreciation of where your patient is at, the next step is to choose an appropriate method.

2. Knowledge and use of appropriate methods

(principles 1, 2, 5, 6 and 7)

Methods are the different ways of applying homeopathy that have developed over the past 200 years. A homeopath will have a good understanding of these methods and be able to choose the most appropriate one for their individual patient. Choosing the most appropriate method of applying homeopathy will make the patient easier to cure.

Chapter 3 will concentrate on bringing you up to date with the variety of methods used, in some form, by today's homeopaths. It doesn't promote a particular method but gives you an easy to follow guide to the methods available.

3. Appropriate use of a repertory

A repertory is an index, list or catalogue. It provides a means of accessing the materia medica without having to compare endless lists of symptoms. It allows a short list to be drawn up that can then be further studied in order to select the most effective remedy. The repertory was introduced into homeopathy because the growth of materia medicas made it difficult to find the appropriate remedy easily. It offers a bridge between the patient's case and the remedy picture in the materia medica and it should be seen as a complementary tool to the materia medica. A repertory is one of the homeopath's most valuable tools.

4. Appropriate use of a therapeutics book

A therapeutics book is a specialised materia medica that links individual diseases with remedies that are known to be effective with a particular disease. It allows you to give remedies that will directly match the disorder and bring relief (but may not fit the constitutional type of the patient). Usually when selecting remedies, several remedies may seem well indicated and it is important at this point to get clear where the disease is coming from in order to differentiate between them.

5. Appropriate use of a materia medica

The words 'materia medica' come from the Latin word 'mater' meaning materials and 'medica' which refers to its use in medicine. Hahnemann created the first *Materia Medica Pura* – 'the book of pure medicine'. Since then homeopaths have developed many more.

They usually list substances found naturally in nature. The vast majority of remedies come from the plant and mineral kingdom. But some materia medicas will have provings of the nosodes (diseased tissues) and drug pictures such as cortisone and penicillin.

Essentially a materia medica is a book on toxicology which records of the effects of poisons on human beings – ie a proving. This record is the basis of a remedy picture. This is supported by clinical experience which adds to the development of the picture.

Materia medicas are often seen as being the essence of homeopathy, when in fact they are a just another tool to be used at the right time and right place. This is the last place you go to and you should only go to it once you have analysed and evaluated the case and are clear what needs to be cured.

6. The 'laws' of homeopathy.

There are a number of 'laws' of homeopathy that are important for you to understand. These 'laws' have been developed by eminent homeopaths based on their own experience. As with any science they are open to question and reinterpretation over time.
The key ones are:

- Principle of similars
- Doctrine of drug proving
- Theory of vital force
- Law of minimum dose
- Law of simplex
- Theory of chronic disease
- Doctrine of drug-dynamisation
- Hering's 'law of cure'.

I don't intend to go into all of these, but you should be aware of them and their place in homeopathy.

For our purposes Hering's 'law of cure' provides a very useful tool of observation. It helps you know your treatment strategy is working as your patients cases unfold in reverse order to how they got sick. Although Hahnemann had the original idea about a 'law of cure', it was Constantine Hering who developed the concept and proposed a useful set of guidelines for homeopaths.

Hering's 'law of cure'

Cures proceed from above downward: symptoms should be seen to move from above downwards as the patient's health improves. This is clearly seen with skin disorders, such as eczema, where the original symptoms improve but they move further down the trunk to the lower limbs (for example a patient with facial eczema could expect the face to clear up but symptoms to appear lower down the body as the cure progresses).

From within outward: symptoms should move outwards from internal organs towards the skin. This can be seen when arthritic joint problems disappears – but a rash appears on the body.

From the most important organ to the least important organ: one of the most important directions is that health should improve in a more important organ and move into a less important organ, for example from asthma in the lungs to eczema on the skin.

In reverse order to the appearance of the symptoms: the disease process should heal in reverse order to the way it started. This can be clearly observed when studying a patient's time-line. For example, practitioners will often observe that a specific emotional aetiology (such as the death of a loved one) has a time lapse of several years before physical symptoms (such as asthma) appear.

However, when they start treating the asthma it is likely that all the emotions of grief start to surface and the lungs will begin to function better. Generally the last symptoms of the disease to appear are the most serious and are likely to relate to deeper pathology, suppression and a chronic state. Usually, as the body heals, these are the symptoms that disappear first, while earlier, less serious, symptoms reappear.

Hering's law will help you evaluate the remedy reaction and give you guidance when observing how your patients are doing. It is important to understand this is a process of healing and the disease is not getting worse! Patients will need to be supported during this process to help them understand what's happening.

Other health practitioners, such as naturopaths, nutritionists and cranial-sacral therapists, are adopting these 'laws' because they are based on observation and experience.

These laws will guide you to look at your patient's symptoms within the context of the cause of those symptoms.

7. Understanding of nutrition and herbal tinctures

Nowadays nutrition and herbal tinctures are an essential support when you are working with patients.

Today's patients are often nutritionally depleted and extremely toxic. People can't be expected to heal if they don't have the basic building blocks to do so. At best nothing will happen, at worst they will really aggravate and you may never see them again. You don't need to do a nutritional course but you can guide them with good common sense suggestions. This is what is called adjunctive advice, it is not homeopathy but it will support your treatment programme, and empower your patients to help themselves.

The issue is in the tissue
Anon

Summary

Homeopathy and allopathy have a fundamentally different approach to dealing with health and sickness. Understanding this will help you to see the individuality of your patients and support you in remaining objective.

A working knowledge of the energetic paradigms will help you to understand the underlying science of homeopathy – a science based on empiricism using observation of the human condition over many years and cultures.

Being able to understand anatomy, physiology and pathology from both a western-based allopathic perspective and a wider homeopathic perspective enables you to make use of diagnostic tools used by allopaths. You will begin to observe the damage caused by a long-term reliance on toxic drugs and invasive surgery to prevent disease. You can then develop a treatment strategy to undo this damage and give support to the innate healing mechanism of the vital energy.

Being clear and able to use some of the basic tools of the homeopathic trade will enable you to practice successfully.

The essential tool-kit for the homeopath

- the ability to take a case and a time-line
- knowledge of and appropriate use of methods
- appropriate use of a repertory, a therapeutics book and a materia medica
- knowledge and appropriate use of the 'laws of homeopathy'
- understanding of nutrition and herbal tinctures.

You should now have a grasp of the importance of

- a grounding in the basic principles of homeopathy
- the need for knowledge and understanding of the wider history and philosophy of healing through the ages
- a good working knowledge of anatomy, physiology and pathology from a homeopathic perspective
- knowledge of other energy paradigms
- good powers of observation.

In Chapter 2 we review the fundamentals of case-taking and the art of taking a time-line. This is because with all methods the formulation of an accurate and detailed time-line is invaluable. A time-line organises the patient's case into a manageable format, helping to clarify cause, effect and obstacles to cure. With certain part-patient methods, the time-line is central to the efficacy of the method.

The guiding principles of CAUSE – EFFECTS – and OBSTACLE
TO CURE used by homeopaths in fact apply to all aspects
life – personal, professional and developmental. They ar
universal principles and once you understand this th
study and practice of homeopathy becomes easie

Ellen Krame

Chapter 2

Case taking and the use of time-lines

The essence of achieving a successful outcome for patients from homeopathy is in your ability to observe the patient and ask the right questions. Being able to take a case and make use of a time-line are important skills that you need to develop. This will help you to place the symptoms your patient is giving you into a context. In addition, having a set of guidelines (Hering's law of cure) to help you observe if the patient is getting better or if you are suppressing or palliating symptoms, will ensure that you are able to follow the process of healing and treat accordingly.

The process of arriving at particular remedies is supported by taking a structured and systematic approach.

This is where a good time-line is invaluable and will lead you to choosing the most appropriate method to maximise the curative results of the remedies. The case should be taken without prejudice, bearing in mind both the cause of the symptoms and the context of the presenting symptoms. You also need to have an understanding of what the underlying constitutional state is and have a feel for the vitality and energy level of your patient.

You must become a good observer and an astute evaluator of all that is going on within the patient's time-line. And you need to be able to see the symptoms presented within a deeper and wider context. (Books such as Louis Hay's *You can heal your life* are excellent guides for developing observational skills). The more you understand the physical and emotional symptoms and their possible causes and relate them to basic principles, the better you become at finding (and treating) the obstacles to cure and choosing a method. Developing your powers of observation helps you to ask the right questions and that is the real art of homeopathy!

When looking at a patient's case bear in mind

Cause – effects – and – obstacles to cure

What is CLAMS?

This is a mnemonic that is commonly used by homeopaths to help them to remember that all general symptoms of disease present as one of the following:

C — **Concomitant**: a symptom that occurs simultaneously to the presenting symptom.

L — **Location**: site where the symptom presents, including sides of the body, direction and extension of pain or sensation to other parts.

A — **Aetiology**: the event or factor that caused the onset of the symptom.

M — **Modalities**: factors that affect the symptom, for better or worse, eg temperature, environment, weather, times of day, motion or action of the remedy, right or left.

S — **Sensations**: Descriptive feeling of symptom for example throbbing, burning, hot or chilly.

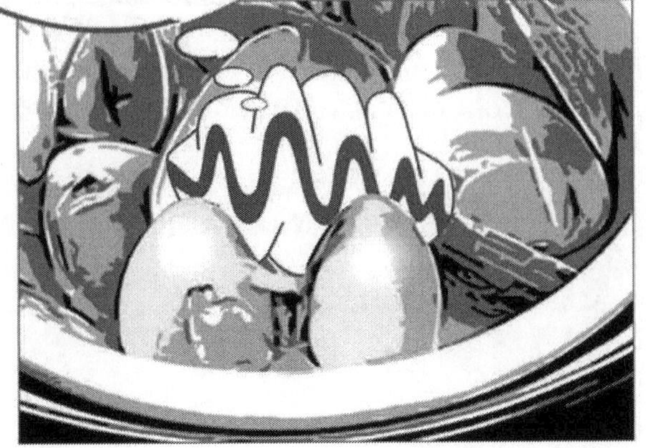

Case-taking

1. Name, address and contact details

Ask the patient what they want or expect from homeopathic treatment.

2. The patient

- a brief description of the patient
- any relevant medical and family histories
- where do they live, and who with.

Be aware of your first impressions of the patient and any assumptions that you initially make about them.

3. A brief overview of the presenting symptoms

For example headache, mood swings or fever – take as given. This will help you decide if it is an acute or chronic case. Don't forget to ask them how old they were when the symptoms started.

4. Physical symptoms

Most patients will have some physical pain that has driven them to consult you. If the patient is in pain fill out your symptom picture by exploring:

- how different positions and motion affect the pain
- if the complaint or the person are worse or better at any particular time or times for example < 5am or 4–8pm
- history of physical traumas. Drug history (legal and leisure).

Then take the physical symptoms starting from head to toe. **Remember CLAMS.**

Head and neck: headaches, concussions, scalp conditions. Trouble at the top of the spine or base of the skull should be put with the head.

Eyes, ears, nose and mouth: styes, conjunctivitis, sticky eyes, earache, sinusitis, hay fever, abscesses, ulcers, cold sores, gum boils, teeth problems.

Throat, chest, lungs and heart: regular sore throats, pain and constriction in the chest, difficulty breathing, palpitations, pain.

Digestive system: heaviness and discomfort after eating, indigestion, bloating, nausea or vomiting.

Abdomen: liver, spleen, kidneys, intestines, colon.

Rectum: haemorrhoids, fissures, bleedings, itching, oozing, pains and constipation.

Urination: any difficulties, pain, discomforts. Frequency and times. Deposits, clear or cloudy, hot, if urination > or <. General changes in its nature, including colour and smell.

Sexual libido and organs:
Male: discharges, disabilities, history of STD and desires.
Female: menses, regularity, PMT, pain, history of contraception and their hormonal history.

Back: pains, aches, sore spots and disabilities.

Skin: sweat – average, above average, below average (for that person), eruptions, and effects of contact with toxic materials.

Energy: too much, too little, just right, ask for a percentage.

5. General Symptoms

- Daily habits and routines: cleanliness, exercise, nutrition and diet, specific stimulants – tea, coffee, alcohol, drugs, smoking.
- Are they generally affected by seasons, weather or temperature.
- Physical sensations: the more unusual the better. For example: *'sensation of warm air steaming up spine into head'*.
- Sleep patterns – nightmares and recurring dreams.

Their answers or lack of answers to these questions will lead you to wider-ranging questions. For example – how they react to heights, how they feel at the seaside or in the mountains, when do they feel like fainting or how they react to tight collars, belts or tight clothing. These questions should be prompted by something the patient has already said!

6. Mental and emotional symptoms

Ask about their general mental and emotional well-being:

- Their occupation past and present, any specific stresses.
- Their relationships with their family, partner, friends and work colleagues.

Ask them how their friends would describe them.

Check for:

- Fears and phobias.
- Anger – humiliation, resentment, loss of control, guilt, jealousy.

Ask what was the worst thing that ever happened to them, and when. For example deaths, break-ups, griefs, betrayals, loss of independence, rape or terminations. Be sensitive, it may be wise to build a relationship with them before you go into this!

Always look for the outstanding, unusual or recently changed symptoms since some mental symptoms are always present.

Don't worry if you don't get everything in one session. Be sensitive to the patient, building rapport with them is more important at the beginning! Some subjects, such as sexual history, can be very sensitive, so follow homeopathic principles and don't go too deep too soon!

Dr Elmiger, a Swiss homeopath, developed a new, causally-based view and treatment of chronic illness within homeopathy called 'sequential therapy'.
By careful observation and experimentation in the Hahnemannian tradition, he came to the conclusion that to cure, one had to address the causes. He believes that this can only be done by treating each cause in the reverse order of its occurrence. He also discovered that as an event receded into the past it lost much of its individuality.

Dr Eizayaga, MD (1924–2001) is best known in the UK as the founder of the layers approach. He proposed that a 'constitutional medicine' is prescribed primarily according to a person's genetic endowment and some of the person's deeply-seated psychological tendencies.
A 'fundamental medicine' is prescribed according to the functional symptoms which represent the organism's response to the various stresses it is experiencing. Dr Eizayaga noted that fundamental states may change and pile up on each other like concentric skins of an onion. He also differentiated the treatment of organic pathology from constitutional or fundamental states. He was president of the Argentinian Medical Homoeopathic Association.

Time-lines as case management tools

Life is full of risks, accidents and emotional trauma – fear, anger, humiliation, loss, rejection. Everyone reacts differently to these traumas and as a consequence will present with different symptoms of stress at various levels of severity.

From a homeopathic perspective the vital energy is designed to maintain balance and is part of the innate healing mechanism. So it is not so much the force of the 'shock' that is important, but the strength of the person's vital energy to overcome it.

Homeopathic treatment is designed to support the vital energy in its efforts to keep a person healthy and to maintain homeostasis.

Through clinical experience and observation it is clear that

- The vital energy becomes weaker with each successive generation if the true cause of disease is not addressed. This is especially true with a history of vaccinations, the abuse of steroids and the use of synthetic oestrogens. This level of suppression can be seen as part of the miasmatic inheritance of modern children.

- The drastic rise in allopathic drug and surgical intervention, as a method of suppression, can lead to long-term chronic illness and serious consequences for the individual because they can be a shock to the vital energy.

- Natural childhood diseases play a vital role in maturing the immune system, but if they are suppressed by vaccination and/or drugs it can be a shock to the vital energy. This is especially true of people who are nutritionally deficient or immune-compromised.

Shocks and traumas

Dr Elmiger suggests that a broad generalisation is that 20% of disease states come as a result of physical shocks and traumas such as:

Pre-birth (miasmic inheritance): the emotional or physical state of the mother during gestation, including any drugs she is taking, must be taken into consideration when treating a child. Most of us carry some biological baggage with us and so the family medical history is important to the extent that heart, liver, respiratory, digestive problems run in the family. Drugs, cigarettes, alcohol, accidents, exhaustion or severe illnesses (especially viral infections) during gestation will have a knock-on effect on the vitality of a child.

Birth: difficult and prolonged labour, induced labour, use of forceps, induction, possible oxygen deprivation, caesarean sections. Insufficient shaping of the baby's head during contractions, anaesthetics (epidural), pain-killing drugs, incubators, blood transfusions, vitamin K injections etc. These shocks may be experienced by the mother too.

Natural childhood illnesses: if children have been weakened by poor nutrition, abuse of antibiotics, artificial hormones, or a vaccination programme – childhood illnesses such as chickenpox, measles and rubella may not be dealt with properly and so fail to carry out their natural function of strengthening the child's immune response.

Vaccinations: too many at one time and/or too soon. Long-term effects of MMR and the pertussis vaccine can remove the ability of the immune system to mature. Travel vaccinations can also have severe side-effects.

Accidents: all kinds, especially external impact injuries, concussion and spinal injuries.

Surgical interventions and major dental work: any kind of surgical procedure, minor or major.

Heavy or prolonged use of drugs: antibiotics, anti-depressants, painkillers, cortisone, birth control pill, HRT, recreational drugs, alcohol, gold salts, and stimulants. Many drug and alcohol abusers are in a permanent state of shock.

Severe viral infections: for example Lyme's disease, mononucleosis, Epstein-Barr virus, measles, chickenpox or mumps.

Serious diseases: sexually transmitted diseases, malaria, tuberculosis, mononucleosis, typhoid, cholera and hepatitis.

Miscellaneous: electric shock therapy and lightning.

Environmental: exposure to toxicity from heavy metals and poisons.

Diet: poor diet rich in refined carbohydrates, excessive consumption of processed foods and nutritional deficiencies.

Dr Elmiger also believes that around 80% of disease states came as a result of mental or emotional shocks and traumas such as:

Loss: deaths, relationship break-ups, job loss, loss of trust, betrayal, loss of childhood and loss of independence.

Fear: prolonged states of fear due to emotional or physical abuse and neglect. Events that leave a person feeling powerless and frightened.

Traumas: involving abuse whether mental, emotional or sexual, particularly in childhood.

Suppressed anger: indignation, humiliation, resentment, guilt and loss of control over life.

Jealousy, envy: sibling rivalry, job promotion and relationship issues.

Unresolved conflicts: that leave a person feeling powerless.

Belief systems: especially strongly-held family belief systems that promote negativity, low self-esteem.

Using a time-line to record the sequence of events leading up to the presenting symptoms is a useful shortcut to help you to see the root causes of disease.

A typical example of a time-line

33 year old woman Presenting symptoms: constipation, irregular menses, headaches.	
Age	**Event**
0	Caesarean birth – her parents thought she would be a boy. They were disappointed. All childhood vaccinations.
2	Brother was born. Her parents doted on him. She had bad temper tantrums and was very jealous of him.
5–11	At school her parents compared her to her brother. She was diagnosed with dyslexia. She feels that she has always had to work harder then anyone else to achieve anything.
12	Onset of menses, painful and irregular.
14	Put on the pill for irregular menses. Put on weight, especially on breasts. She feels she's never lost it.
16	Left school.
17	Started a job, had sex with the boss and had to move jobs.
20	Brother went to university. Her parents were very proud of him.
21	Heavy binge drinking. Regularly smoked cannabis. Most of her money was spent on drugs. Frequent hangovers.
25	Promoted at work. Irritable bowel syndrome (IBS) started. Irregular sleep as she worried about deadlines. Waking at 3am. Suffered from chronic impacted faeces, hospitalised, more drugs given. Brother graduated from law school.
27	Lots of pressure at work. Out partying most nights, drinking even more.
30	Pregnant although still on the pill, termination.
31–33	Stopped the pill. Irregular menses. Headaches after drinking. Chronic constipation, she's lucky to go once a week. When her father died she felt sad that she never got to know him well.

Using time-lines

A time-line is a clearly recorded list of the patient's health history including any problems and significant life events. It should be in chronological order. This is easier to do at the second appointment after you've reviewed their previous prescription.

Guide the patient through the following process

Map out at what age their symptoms first occurred. Each key 'event' is identified and put in chronological order using five or seven year cycles, for example 'what happened in your life between birth to five years, and so on until the present day?'.

Ask them to tell you their reaction to the event whether physical, mental or emotional, and if they have ever felt this way before or since. Always use their language, if they felt 'pissed off' then write that down. This will probably take about 30-40 minutes, you will have to keep focused and manage the time, particularly if the patient is a 'talker' or a 'rambler'. At the end, check

- have they told you everything they think is important?
- have you asked them everything you think is important?

Be aware that states can change and tend to become more physical over time, so it can take up to two to five years (or longer) before physical symptoms appear after mental, emotional shocks and traumas. So if they give you a symptom, always ask them what was happening in their lives prior to the symptoms coming on.

Summary

Using your patient's time-line as a case management tool will help you develop the bigger picture and enhance your ability to find the most appropriate method as a prescribing tool.

Note to what extent the following have played a part

- probable causes and recurring patterns, (because this will give you an understanding of how their vital energy reacts to events of life)
- whether specific 'events' may have played a role
- the activity of the miasms
- the level of toxicity in the case, and any maintaining causes and the extent to which initial palliation may be necessary
- how strong the vital energy of the patient appears to be.

Two of the key questions to ask are

- what caused the trauma? *and*
- are there any obstacles to cure?

These two questions will help you decide what the most appropriate method is for this patient.

Correctly identifying these shocks and traumas at an early stage in the treatment process is a key part of the successful homeopath's skill and will help immeasurably in clarifying what is needed to bring about a cure. It is important that homeopaths not only understand the importance of using a time-line but learn to do so quickly and effectively.

This process is invaluable as it will help you choose the most appropriate method of applying homeopathy in order to help the patient to cure. (*Principle 2 – Healing should be accomplished in the most speedy, gentle and reliable manner*).

You should now have a grasp of the importance of

- good case-taking skills
- an understanding of the use of time-lines as case management tools.

In the next chapters we concentrate on giving a comprehensive update on the methods that have been developed over time by different schools of thought in homeopathy. In essence they are all methods developed by homeopaths looking for ways to deal with patient's disease.

The only thing that is ever true in homeopathy is a cured patient – everything else is just the method of applying homeopathy to achieve a cure.

Robert Davidson

Chapter 3

Methods: introduction to the general concepts

The Chambers dictionary describes a method as 'the mode or rule used in carrying out a task or accomplishing an aim; an orderly procedure'.

'Methods' are the different ways of applying homeopathy that have been developed over the past 200 years. You need to have a good understanding of these and be able to choose the most appropriate one for your patient. It is very limiting to think that a system of medicine should only be applied in one way. I suspect that is why Hahnemann spent his time writing and rewriting the Organon. The body does not do symptoms for the sake of it, there is always a reason even if it is obscure and hidden. The answer lies in the case, not in our opinion of how we should apply homeopathy. Homeopathy is not a religion but a system of medicine. It must evolve to keep up with the types of disease and the effects of the levels of suppression caused by allopathic treatment.

A homeopath should have a good working knowledge of the principles behind each method and be able to use the appropriate method for each patient. (*Principles 1, 2, 5, 6 and 7*).

It is pointless arguing that one method is better than another. Your patients won't care what method you use, all they are interested in is the result. If you are not getting the results with your chosen method – try another and see if it works.

You should now be aware of the usefulness of taking a clear case and establishing a time-line for each individual patient. As already said, one of the most effective ways of choosing a method is to take a time-line and use it as a case management tool. This effectively gives you an overview of how your patient moved from health into pathology.

Methods are the many different ways of applying homeopathy. They are ways of approaching the same problem – that of prescribing the most effective remedies. The different methods use different styles and place a slightly different emphasis on the varying factors that are important to bear in mind when prescribing homeopathically.

Choosing a method

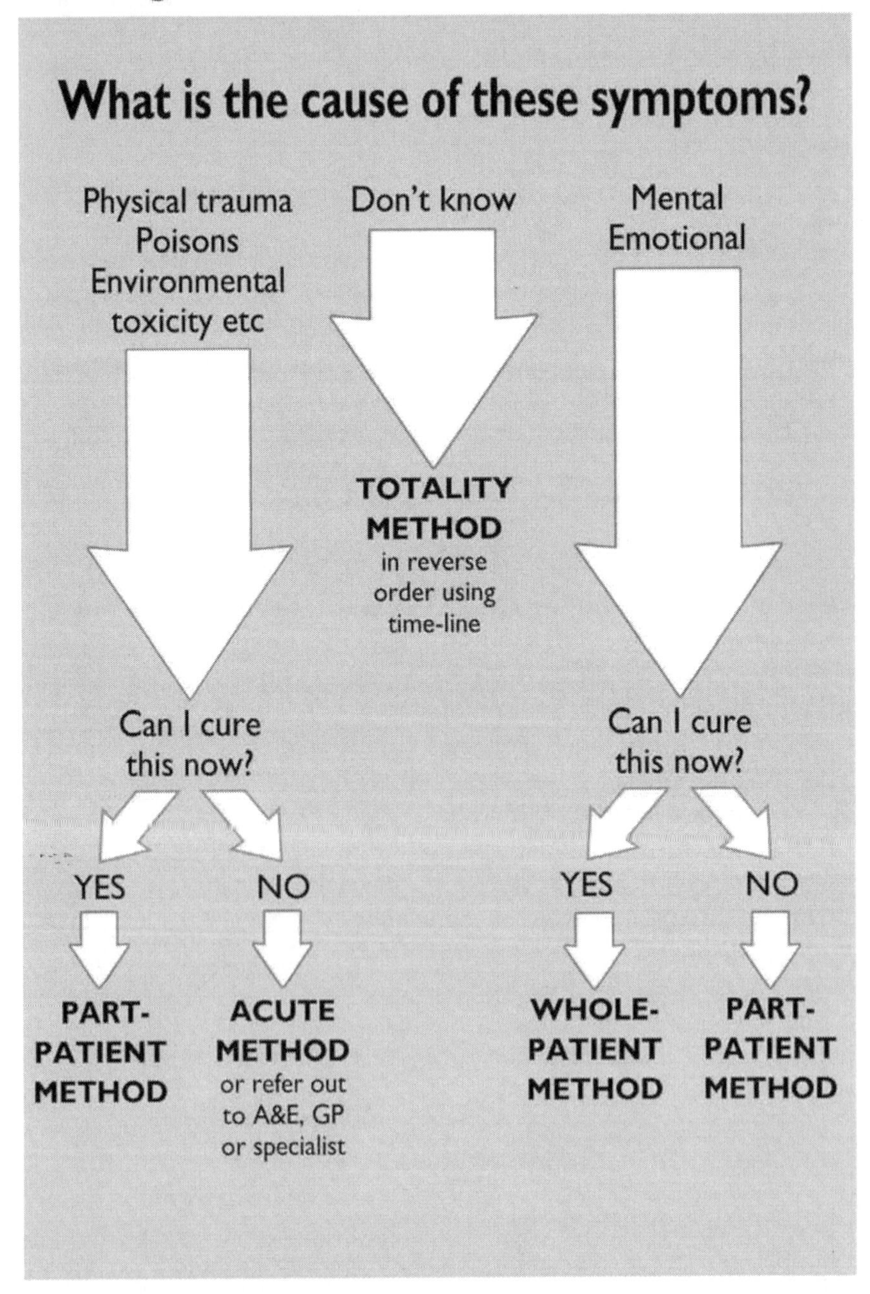

Having gained an appreciation of where your patient is at, you can move on to choosing an appropriate method.
(Principle 2: healing should be accomplished in the most speedy, gentle and reliable manner)
To be able to choose a method you need to understand the context of the symptoms the patient is presenting. Samuel Hahnemann said: 'Every homeopath must have a good understanding of what causes and sustains illness and how to eliminate it from healthy people'.

If you put the basic principles of homeopathy (see Chapter 1) into practice and return to them if confused, they will act as an anchor to keep you linked to the underlying philosophy of homeopathy.

A wide understanding of other healing paradigms and a good basic knowledge of anatomy, physiology and pathology from a homeopathic perspective will help you avoid becoming a remedy chaser, using increasing more esoteric methods of guessing the remedy, or being tempted to use remedies as alternatives to allopathic drugs (which appears to be increasingly common among some homeopaths). Given the diversity of symptoms and of the remedies available, a practical shortcut must be developed – hence the need for a good time-line and for repertorisation techniques.

A useful way to learn and apply methods is to classify them into two main groups

Whole-patient methods: there are five main whole-patient methods. These focus on the person and disease symptoms that come out of mental or emotional causations. The disease symptoms are usually functional in nature (for example constipation, asthma, tinnitus or vertigo). Whole-patient methods consider symptoms and characteristics relative to the person and the disease simultaneously.

Part-patient methods: these consider symptoms and the person's characteristics relative to the disease only. These tend to focus on disease symptoms that have some kind of tissue change, obstacles to cure, organ dysfunction, physical trauma or poisonings. Part-patient methods all produce a therapeutic prescription of one form or another. These therapeutic prescriptions are all achieved and styled differently according to what is perceived to be the disease or pathology in need of curing.

More explanation will be given to the layers method, which you will notice, features in both groups.

Choosing a method

On first analysis of a case, you must perceive what needs curing and decide whether your approach will involve a whole-patient method or a part-patient method or a combination of them both.

With all methods the formulation of an accurate time-line is invaluable because of the need to place symptoms in the correct context. A detailed time-line organises the patient's case into a manageable format, helping to clarify the cause, effect and need for cure. With certain part-patient methods, the time-line is central to the efficacy of the method.

All methods produce a prescription which is individual to the patient. Methods help you focus on the most important symptoms in the case.

It is important to ask yourself a series of questions to help you choose a method. You may need to combine two different methods and develop a treatment strategy: this is often necessary if patients are very ill and on multiple drugs.

Summary

An understanding of the main methods is a fundamental part of your development as a homeopath. The following chapters give a broad description of each of the main methods in current use. This is intended as a general guide and all of the methods presented have a history and a variety of adherents who will have slightly different approaches to that method. Further research is advised – a good place to start is Ian Watson's book (see bibliography). This will give you a deeper insight into the history of each method and point you to original material. Ally this with a good internet search engine and you have the best homeopathic library in the world at your fingertips.

All the methods have their limitations, but by understanding the different methods you can begin to be creative. This ensures that homeopathy continues to grow, develop and evolve to meet the ever increasing levels of suppression and toxicity that our modern twenty-first century patients will present.

Classical homeopathy, which is a single method approach, has its place and context for use, just as a tautopathic approach has its appropriate use in practice. If you are taught to look at patients from one perspective with only one tool in your tool-kit the results will be limited.

The division into two groups is designed to help you to learn and understand the differences between methods, and to help you to be clear what strategy you are using.

There are a number of other approaches to choosing remedies that are currently taught and used by practitioners. I have not addressed these in this guide as I feel they are not sufficiently developed within an empirical scientific framework – for example dream provings, meditation provings, doctrine of signatures, and psychic approaches (pendulum, tarot etc). Nor have I covered iridology, kinesiology, facial diagnosis or the use of QX machines as these are diagnostic tools and not methods. I will give a brief overview of these in Chapter 7.

You should now have a grasp of the importance of

- how a knowledge of the main methods developed so far can be used to assist in the choice of treatment
- how the two main classifications – whole-patient methods and part-patient methods help in choosing the appropriate method for each case
- understanding the classification is not a pecking order of importance but merely for ease of study leading to practical application
- methods as an important part of a homeopath's tool-kit that work alongside the use of a time-line, repertory and materia medica.

In the next chapter we review the five whole-patient methods. These consider symptoms and characteristics relative to the person *and* the disease simultaneously.

The un-tuned vital force causes disease and health is restored when we tune the vital force.

Samuel Hahnemann

Chapter 4

Whole-patient methods

Whole-patient methods consider the spiritual, mental, emotional and physical levels of a patient. They work on the philosophy that the disease process starts from disturbances in the vital energy and then appear as physical symptoms of disease. The cause of the disease generally comes from a mental or emotional cause such as loss, grief, anger, jealousy, humiliation, fear, abuse, unresolved conflicts or belief systems.

Whole-patient methods tend to focus on the person and disease symptoms that come out of mental or emotional causes. The disease symptoms are usually functional in nature, for example constipation, asthma, tinnitus or vertigo. Whole-patient methods consider symptoms and characteristics relative to the person *and* the disease simultaneously.

Each method in this category involves discerning the relevant symptoms of the case and ordering them according to their importance. We describe this as the hierarchy of symptoms. Each method in this group has a different hierarchy of symptoms, which are critical to distinguishing the methods and subsequent prescriptions from one another.

The main whole-patient methods

1. Classical.

2. Totality.

3. Physical generals.

4. Miasmatic.

5. Layers.

This is not a pecking order of importance but merely for ease of study and reading.

1. Classical method

Kentian or constitutional prescribing method

This method treats disease by prescribing on the patient's predominant mental and emotional state. The diseases tend to come from mental or emotional causes and the symptoms tend to manifest as functional disorders such as hayfever or menstrual problems. (It is sometimes called the **Kentian** method but Kent himself called it **constitutional** prescribing).

This method was developed by Kent and marked a transition from taking all symptoms as important (totality prescribing) to placing greater emphasis on symptoms of a mental and emotional level. Before the 1900s this had not been the case. The classical method was a new development and a departure from previous methods.

Symptoms in order of importance

1. Mental and emotional symptoms (including delusions).

2. Physical general symptoms (CLAMS).

3. Physical particular symptoms (disease symptoms).

Notes:

• When deciding what symptoms to repertorise, be sure to include those which are relevant to what you are curing (the cause of the symptoms) and wherever possible, characteristic of the person. In this way you can distinguish what makes Bobby's asthma different from Billy's and so on.

• Where there is a strange, rare or peculiar symptom (SRP) of any sort in the case, this is always considered to be of primary importance when selecting symptoms.

Repertorisation

A standard approach for classical repertorisation involves selecting around eight rubrics from the case in total. Being selective in your choice of symptoms for use as rubrics is an essential discipline, as patients will often bombard you with lots of symptoms which are often confusing and not very helpful.

1. Mental and emotional symptoms 5 rubrics
2. Physical general symptoms 2 rubrics
3. Physical particular symptoms 1 rubric

Appropriate times to use this method

Bold indicates what must be present for this method to be the best choice

- **When the causes of the symptoms are mental or emotional traumas.**
- **When mental or emotional symptoms predominate in the case.**
- When there is no deep pathology.
- When there is no long-term drug layer or clear link between a drug and the presenting complaint.
- In chronic and acute cases.

Prescription guidelines

A single dose, a split dose (two doses, twelve hours apart), or a collective single dose (three doses, each twelve hours apart). Some practitioners repeat this dose (weekly or fortnightly) to counteract the reduction in efficacy caused by environmental toxicity, diet, atmospheric pollution, drugs etc.

2. Totality method
or symptom similarity method

Totality, or symptom similarity, implies finding all the symptoms in the case and matching them to a similar remedy. This could be a difficult and unwieldy process so the key is in how we select symptoms.

Symptom selection

The is simplified by only looking at those symptoms that are:
Strange, rare and peculiar: symptoms are considered strange or rare when they are outside what we would normally expect in that person. Remember to ask yourself 'what is strange about this person's presentation of disease?' Symptoms only become strange, rare and peculiar within the context of the person in whom they are found. This is a very subjective thing but is valuable because you can distinguish individuality clearly and quickly in a case.

Characteristic: these symptoms represent individuality. They distinguish those things that are common to everyone from those that are unique to the individual. They are important because they help us to determine what is different about Sarah's headache from Simon's headache.

These are both related to the individual. You can also use
Keynotes: these are symptoms that are strongly related to a particular remedy picture and often become what we remember most about that remedy for example:

- delusions that rags are beautiful: sulphur
- symptoms are better for motion: rhus-tox
- discharges are thick and ropy: kali-bich
- ailments from bad news: gelsemium

Symptoms in order of importance

Strange, rare and peculiar (SRP) symptoms are the most important symptom within their particular group (ie mental and emotional, physical general and/or physical particular symptoms) and are followed by all other characteristic and keynote symptoms. Use as many as the case offers but it is not necessary to exceed nine in total.

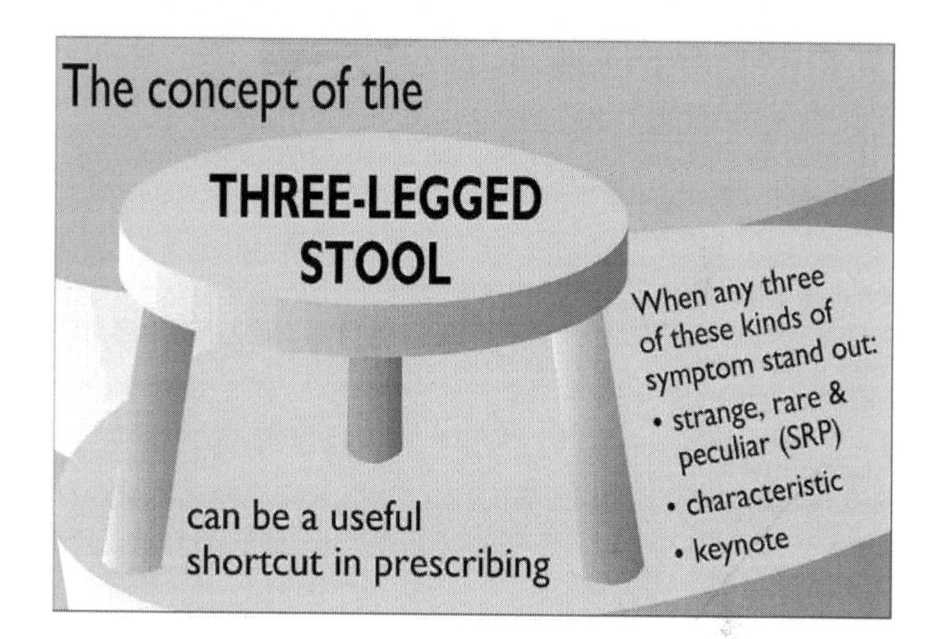

Repertorisation

No formal repertorisation is required. If a remedy is not obvious from the symptoms then cross-referencing the key rubrics is a way of clarifying which is the most indicated remedy.

Appropriate times to use this method

Bold indicates what must be present for this method to be the best choice

- **When the cause of the symptoms are mental or emotional traumas.**
- When keynote, characteristic and/or SRP symptoms predominate in the case.
- When there is no deep pathology.
- When there is no long-term drug layer or clear link between a drug and the presenting complaint.
- In chronic and acute cases.

Prescription guidelines

Prescriptions are between 30c and CM or LM. Repetition may vary depending on the case.

3. Physical generals method

This method treats disease by prescribing on the patient's predominant physical general symptoms. It is a variation of the classical method, but the emphasis is on the general physical symptoms.

A physical general symptom is when a physical symptom relates to the patient as a whole (such as body temperature) or when the nature of a symptom, such as a throbbing pain, affects more than one single part, creating a theme through the body, for example, throbbing pain in eye, ear, arm and leg.

The main advantage of this method is that you don't have to make a psychological analysis, with all its attendant problems, but can keep to what the physical body is telling you. It requires the prescriber to use the outstanding symptoms in the case and encourages them to make connections between isolated symptoms in the physical body as a whole.

Symptom selection

As with the classical method, symptom selection needs to include those which are relevant to what's being cured and wherever possible, characteristic of the person. Where there is a strange, rare or peculiar symptom (SRP) of any sort in the case, this is always considered to be of primary importance.

All physical general symptoms present as one of these

The first five are commonly known as CLAMS – see chapter 3.

Concomitant: a symptom that occurs at the same time as the presenting symptom.

Location: the site where the symptom presents, including sides of the body, direction and extension of pain or sensation to other parts.

Aetiology: the event or factor that caused the onset of the symptom.

Modalities: factors that affect the symptom, for example, are they better(>) or worse (<) for: temperature, environment, weather, times of day or motion.

Sensations: descriptive feeling of the symptom, such as throbbing, burning, hot, chilly.

Food: strong desires, aversions or responses to food and drink Appetite and thirst.

Menses: symptoms relating to cycle, duration, intensity and appearance of flow. Pain and ailments before, during and/or after.

Sleep, dreams: symptoms of disturbance, times of waking, insomnia and nightmares.

Sexual: symptoms of libido and sexual function.

Observable: symptoms and signs of patient's pallor, expression and demeanour.

Repertorisation

About eight rubrics are selected from the case:

1. Physical general symptoms	5 rubrics
2. Mental and emotional symptoms	2 rubrics
3. Physical particular symptoms	1 rubric

Phatak's Concise Repertory has only physical general and particular symptoms and is ideal for this method.

Appropriate times to use this method

Bold indicates what must be present for this method to be the best choice

- **When the cause of the symptoms is mental or emotional traumas**, but physical general symptoms predominate in the case.
- When mental or emotional symptoms are insufficient, unremarkable or unobtainable.
- When there is no deep pathology.
- When there is no long-term drug layer or clear link between a drug and the presenting complaint.
- In chronic and acute cases.

Prescription guidelines

Prescriptions are between 30c and CM. Repetition may vary depending on the case.

4. Miasmatic method

This method involves prescribing on symptoms resulting from dominant miasmatic activity.

Symptom selection

All symptoms characteristic of the dominant miasm are of equal importance. It is not always the symptom picture of the case that is prescribed upon using this method. See the layers method (next) for more information on miasmatic prescribing.

Repertorisation

No formal repertorisation is required though cross-referencing the key rubrics is a way of clarifying which is the indicated nosode, if recognition from symptoms is not obvious.

Appropriate times to use this method

- In chronic and acute cases.
- When the nosode is the indicated remedy based on the presenting symptom picture.
- When the indicated remedy fails to act or cure
- When the symptom picture is unclear and too mixed up to fathom.
- When the action of an indicated remedy doesn't hold and the state relapses.
- When acute states don't resolve with the indicated remedy and become sub-acute or chronic states.
- As an intercurrent throughout layers prescribing – a miasmatic prescription given at selected intervals during the treatment with the indicated remedy.

Prescription guidelines

Prescriptions are commonly between 30c and 10M and are given as either a single dose or with more frequent repetition, for example intercurrently.

5. Layers method

This method helps you to prescribe within a logical and ordered structure. The case is organised into a series of layers. It is the only method that combines whole-patient and part-patient approaches. You use a whole-patient method when you look at the case from the fundamental layer and a part-patient method when you look at the case from the drug and lesion layers. Each layer is treated within a structured sequence as seen below. The miasm layer runs like a thread through the other layers.

Traditionally the use of this method requires you to access the case from either the drug or lesion layer depending on the amount of drug toxicity or pathology the patient presents. Prescribing the appropriate remedies should lead to the case unravelling in reverse order to the process of becoming sick and eventually taking the patient back to their original constitutional state.

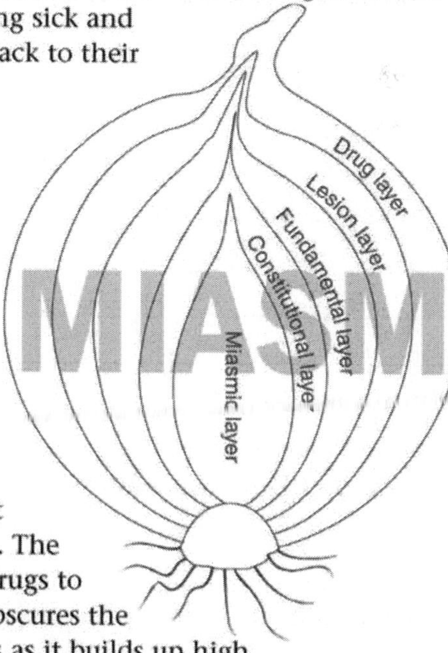

The layers are:

- Drug layer.
- Lesion layer.
- Fundamental layer.
- Constitutional layer.
- Miasmatic layer.

The drug layer

These days it is rare to see a case of pathology that does not have a drug layer of some kind. The long-term use of prescription drugs to suppress specific pathologies obscures the true picture of a disease process as it builds up high levels of toxicity in the system and causes many side-effects. Due to the impact of this on key organs (such as the liver and kidneys) it can act as an obstacle to cure by interfering with or undermining the effect of remedies to bring about a cure. Therefore this layer is treated before the pathology itself by way of a detox therapeutic prescription. When the drug layer has been cleared, the lesion layer (pathology) is treated.

The lesion layer

A lesion is classified when disease or pathology has localised in a system, organ or tissue. The lesion layer (within the layers method) refers to disease of a chronic nature and is treated by a lesion therapeutic prescription. This will utilise all symptoms relative to the disease only.

The symptoms associated with the lesion are repertorised with the disease rubric being the most important. This is because the indicated remedy will be found in the Repertory under the name of the disease. Other relevant rubrics will help to differentiate the disease state to the individual. The hierarchy of symptoms must state the lesion or pathology rubric first, as well as including any mental and general symptoms that have appeared as a result of the disease. Mental and physical general symptoms are only included if they are part of the lesion, eg if depression is seen as a result of being told they have cancer.

- Physical particular symptoms, including pathology rubric first, for example 'endometriosis' — 5 rubrics
- Physical general symptoms — 2 rubrics
- Mental and emotional symptoms — 1 rubric

The fundamental layer

This layer involves prescribing on the mental and emotional state once symptoms of toxicity and pathology are absent. These symptoms are of a functional nature only and relate to the whole person, not just the process of disease. They are seen as acquired and are a deviation from the patient's naturally healthy state. This layer overlaps with the classical method and uses the same hierarchy of symptoms:

- mental and emotional symptoms (including delusions)
- physical general symptoms (CLAMS)
- physical particular symptoms (disease symptoms).

Fundamental symptoms are not who the patient 'is', they are who the patient has 'become'. When these acquired mental symptoms have been cured, the constitutional layer is treated.

The constitutional layer

In this layer symptoms of the constitution such as colouring, body shape, personality and general modalities are seen as the healthy state of the person and not part of any pathology, nor are they in need of cure. Prescribing at this level is intended to fortify the constitution (basic healthy state) and help maintain good health. The ultimate aim of homeopathy is to return a patient to this level of health.

Dr Eizayaga first named four main constitutional remedies *(but other respected homeopaths have changed it to five by adding silica):*
• calc carb • calc fluor • phosphorous • sulphur • silica.
The indicated constitutional remedy is identified through similarity of characteristic symptoms. All characteristic symptoms are of equal importance.

The miasmatic layer

Traditionally the layers method was structured with the miasmatic layer underneath all the others. Modern day disease requires us to prescribe on the miasmatic layer intercurrently, that is alongside other layers. This is because as symptoms are suppressed miasmatic states will change.

As with the miasmatic method, all symptoms characteristic of the dominant miasm are of equal importance and no formal repertorisation is needed (partly because the nosodes are usually under represented in most repertories). A prescription tends to be reached using the totality of symptoms for the whole patient.

Appropriate times to use this method

Bold indicates what must be present for this method to be the best choice

- **When there is pathology or multiple pathologies with long-term drug use.**
- In chronic cases.

Prescription guidelines

All prescriptions are given in low potency, 6-30c or 6x-30x, with frequent repetition – up to four times daily. Water remedies are often more effective as the energy of the remedy is constantly stimulated by the movement of the water. This is thought to prevent the system from becoming dulled to the remedy's action.

Summary

On the whole these methods focus on symptoms that come out of mental or emotional causations. These methods provide a structured and logical approach for selecting relevant symptoms from what can be a plethora of confusing symptoms from the patient. They work very well with basically healthy constitutions; the type of constitution you will see in rural areas of Africa, South America, India or Indonesia where people are not overly-exposed to suppressive drug treatment and have not transgressed too far from their natural diets.

If 80% of disease comes out of mental or emotional causations then one would expect to use one of the whole-patient methods for 80% of one's practice. Unfortunately modern western patients have been so heavily suppressed that I often find I only use one of these methods for 20% of my practice.

You should now understand that

- the division is not in order of importance but merely for ease of study leading to practical application
- the five whole-patient methods are
  1. Classical
  2. Totality
  3. Physical generals
  4. Miasmatic
  5. Layers
- whole-patient methods consider symptoms and characteristics relative to the person and the disease simultaneously
- whole-patient methods tend to focus on the person *and* the disease symptoms that come out of mental and emotional causations such as loss, grief, anger, jealousy, humiliation, fear, abuse, unresolved conflicts and belief systems
- the disease symptoms are usually functional in nature, for example constipation, asthma, tinnitus, vertigo
- each of the methods in this category involves discerning relevant symptoms of the case and ordering them according to their importance. We describe this as the **hierarchy of symptoms.**

In Chapter 5 we look at the part-patient methods.

Healing is easy if you keep it simple and know what you are doing...so acquire the right tools and learn to apply them like a master. In this way creativity flows and homeopathy grows.

Ellen Kramer

Chapter 5

Part-patient methods

The concept of part-patient methods focuses your attention on the patient's dysfunction, presenting pathology and/or drug history as individual separate issues to be treated in their own context.

The causation of symptoms comes from

- physical shocks and traumas: pre-birth or birth traumas, natural childhood illnesses, accidents, surgical interventions and major dental work, severe viral infections and diseases, or
- drug, environmental toxicity, poor nutrition and diet, organ insufficiency, vaccinations, heavy or prolonged use of drugs (prescribed and lifestyle).

The main part-patient methods

1. Clinical prescribing
2. Acute
3. Aetiological
4. Sequential
5. Isopathic
6. Tautopathic
7. Prophylactic
8. Detox therapeutic

Each of these methods is influenced by the time-line and varies according to the issue or tissue involved.

Part-patient methods are often used to remove obstacles to cure such as organ dysfunction, poor lines of elimination, poisons, poor nutritional states or physical traumas.

Homeopathic approaches to detoxifying patients are often used as part of an overall treatment programme. As well as the detox therapeutic method I have given three other detox approaches commonly used. These are:

- Organ support
- The Singh approach
- Bowel nosode programme

1. Clinical prescribing
or therapeutic method

The emphasis of this method is on treating the disease process rather than the person. The causation of symptoms comes from physical shocks and traumas and organ dysfunction or there is a history of suppression from allopathic medicine. It is especially useful for treating:

- first aid cases
- acute diseases
- chronic levels of toxicity within the system before they develop into pathology
- chronic pathological states.

Symptom selection

This method is extremely effective when individualised because the emphasis is on the physical problem. It does require a certain amount of individualisation of the disease state and its causations. In order to choose the correct strategy, it is important to keep going back to the patients time-line so that you can identify the most effective area to prescribe on therapeutically. This is especially important when using this method in chronic cases.

The main ways of individualisation

- addressing the causes of disease
- detoxification
- supporting key organs.

These are not in a hierarchy and you should choose the most appropriate for your patient.

The art of therapeutic prescribing is knowing the causations and the keynote symptoms of therapeutic remedies for that disease state. The more you practice this method the better you get at selecting the most effective remedy.

There are two ways of choosing a therapeutics remedy

- by using a repertory to find the indicated remedy, or
- by using a therapeutics book.

CLAMS is a useful tool when using this method to help you differentiate between remedies.

Using a repertory to find the indicated remedy

You can repertorise for the therapeutics method by using the following hierarchical order (as in Eizayaga's lesion layer):

1. physical particular symptoms, including pathology rubric first – for example endometriosis	5 rubrics
2. physical general symptoms	2 rubrics
3. mental and emotional symptoms associated with the disease or acute state	1 rubric

Using a therapeutics book

You focus on the totality of disease symptoms and any mental or emotional symptoms that go with the pathology.

First you identify a group of remedies that are known to have a proven clinical relationship to the particular disease process from a therapeutics book This could be your own book developed from experience or a recommended one. Then you select the most appropriate remedy for this particular disease state from the therapeutics book.

Prescription guidelines

There are no restrictions on potency or frequency of repetition with this method.

2. Acute method

This method involves prescribing on a disorder or dysfunction of short duration. This could be anything from a few hours to several days. Acute states that do not resolve within this time-frame become sub-acutes and may well need to be treated with both an acute therapeutic and a miasmatic intercurrent.

The acute state is often severe and intense, requiring immediate, sometimes life-saving, prescribing. The emphasis is placed upon treating the process of the disorder, and not the person. As with all homeopathic prescriptions, the most effective acute therapeutics are those that have been individualised.

Deciding on a remedy involves differentiating between groups of remedies which all have an affinity for the presenting symptoms, using the presenting CLAMS to individualise. See page 18.

Appropriate times to use this method

- For infectious disease.
- In emergency and first aid situations.
- In pregnancy and labour.
- For intense symptoms in response to a homeopathic prescription for chronic disease (an aggravation!)

Prescription guidelines

An acute therapeutic is given in a low or high potency, 6c–CM or LM, with frequent repetition, dependent upon the severity and intensity of symptoms.

Dissolving a pill in water and sipping frequently is an effective way of treating acutes and is known as 'plussing'. Sub-acute states often require an intercurrent nosode, prescribed alongside the acute therapeutic, at a similar potency.

3. Aetiological method

This method involves prescribing on an event, trauma or disease in the patient's past rather than the presenting symptoms of disease. The time-line plays a vital role in the application of this method as it will provide the evidence of the cause and effect, and highlight where there is need for cure. The stronger the evidence, the more effective this method becomes. There is no time limitation, so no matter how long ago the event, disease or trauma occurred, prescribing on the incident can be effective in addressing the onset of symptoms.

Appropriate times to use this method

Bold indicates what must be present for this method to be the best choice

- **When there is clear evidence from the time-line of cause and effect.**
- When the indicated remedy has failed to cure.
- In chronic or acute cases.

Prescription guidelines

An aetiological prescription can be given in moderate to high potencies, 12c–CM or LM.

A general guide is that the further back in the time-line the causative event occurred, the higher the potency prescribed. The lower potencies can be given with more repetition.

A remedy that ties in with the pathology or tissue affinity for the presenting symptoms is more likely to be successful, for example for cancer of the liver (pathology) you could use chelidonium (suppressed anger).

4. Sequential method

This method is a variation on the aetiological method, where there is evidence of a sequence of causative factors (traumas) that have systematically contributed to the patient's current state of disease. It places aetiology over symptomology. It relies entirely on a detailed and well drawn up time-line.

Events that are likely to appear in the time-line

Childhood	Teenage	Adulthood
• trauma in utero: *physical, drugs, or emotional* • birth trauma • weaning and separation • fear/abuse • vaccination • childhood diseases • friendships	• school, exam pressure • puberty • appearance, peer pressure • vaccination • relationships • drugs, alcohol abuse • fear/abuse	• traumatic life events • fear/abuse • long-term prescriptive or recreational drugs • toxicity • serious disease • surgery

Each event is seen as a separate acute episode. Working with the time-line in sequence involves identifying each trauma in the case, beginning with the most recent and working backwards up to the most remote. Sequential therapy proceeds, as the name suggests, in a sequential fashion but in the exact reverse order of the occurrence of the trauma. Each is identified in the case-taking and placed in chronological order. The nature of the traumas and the corresponding remedies that have been proven effective are chosen. The most recent trauma is treated first, then the second most recent, up to the birth trauma, and even those suffered by one or both parents. If there have been two traumas of the same kind, for example two periods of heavy cortisone use, with no traumas in between, then they can be treated as one. Traumas seem to exist along the same space-time continuum.

Appropriate times to use this method

Bold indicates what must be present for this method to be the best choice

- **A case with evidence of a sequence of events (traumas) that have brought about the presenting state.**
- In chronic cases.

Prescription guidelines

A sequence (aetiological) therapeutic is prescribed for each event appropriate to the case and individual. Nosodes and polycrest remedies can be given as required. Some homeopaths will start the case with a sequence of indicated nosodes to clear the miasms.

The remedies follow one another in sequence forming what is essentially just one prescription, for example morning, night, morning.

As with aetiological prescribing, the potency and repetition is determined by the severity and intensity of the patient's response to the trauma at the time. This means that in a sequence of remedies, the potencies may vary considerably.

Sarcodes: remedies made from healthy tissue (for example oophorinum is made from the ovary of a sheep or cow, thyroidinum is made from sheep's thyroid gland).

Nosodes: remedies made from diseased tissue or secretions with the specific bacteria, virus or fungus of that disease (for example tuberculinum is made from tubercular abscess or the glycerine extract of the cultivation of human tubercular bacillius).

Polycrest remedies: a group of remedies that are likely to be prescribed for acute, chronic and constitutional cases. This is because they are well represented in the repertory like sulphur, calc carb, lycopodium, phosphorus and arsenicum. (classical homeopaths usually refer to them as constitutional remedies).

5. Isopathic method

This method involves prescribing a remedy made from something that is known to cause symptoms of the presenting disease in a patient or something that patient is hypersensitive to – such as wheat, milk or pollen.

It may also involve prescribing a remedy made from a product of a disease for someone suffering from that disease, for example the potentised whooping cough mucus (from another person) for a patient with whooping cough. If a patient's own discharge or secretion is given as a remedy (auto nosode), this is known as auto-isopathy and is particularly effective in auto-immune diseases.

When using an isopathic approach you are focusing your attention on either substances that are not necessarily toxic or harmful to other people but seem to be the cause of disorders in this particular patient.

Appropriate times to use this method

Bold indicates what must be present for this method to be the best choice

- **When it is clear what the cause of the symptom is, such as wheat causing abdominal pains.**
- When the indicated remedy has failed to cure.
- In cases where the symptoms of disease match the known aggravations of the substance or factor, without it being present in the case.
- In chronic or acute cases.

Prescription guidelines

An isopathic remedy taken over a period of time is often in a low potency, 6–30c or 6x–30x, as either a single dose or with more frequent repetition.

Alternatively a single high dose or ascending doses, such as 30c, 200c, 1M, 10M over a period of days or weeks, might be given to clear an aetiology, (such as sol for 'never been well since sunburn', or the patient's own discharge or secretion when indicated remedies and nosodes fail to work).

6. Tautopathic method

Tautopathy is a form of Isopathy. The difference between the two methods is that in tautopathy you are focusing on a drug or toxin taken by the patient that appears to have caused the symptoms. A tautopathic therapeutic approach involves prescribing the original toxin or drug in low potency, (usually used after the indicated remedy has been given and failed to cure).

Drugs with certain known side-effects can be prescribed in potency to cure similar symptoms produced by disease (for example Aspartame for brain tumours). A tautopathic remedy can also be prescribed alongside drugs that can't be withdrawn, for example warfarin can be given back in potency while the patient is still on the drug. This appears to minimise the side-effects of the drug. Often patients find they can take less of the drug but still get maximum therapeutic value from it.

Drugs or toxins in potency are often prescribed alongside indicated detox therapeutics, in a triad of other organ support remedies, with effective results.

Appropriate times to use this method

Bold indicates what must be present for this method to be the best choice

- **When a drug or toxin is clearly the cause of disease.**
- When the indicated remedy has failed to cure.
- In cases of drug withdrawal.
- In cases where the symptoms of disease match the known side-effects of a drug.
- In chronic or acute cases

Prescription guidelines

When using the tautopathic method to treat the effects of drugs taken over a period of time the prescription is often in a low potency, 6–30c or 6x–30x, as either a single dose or with more frequent repetition. Alternatively a single high dose or ascending doses, such as 30c, 200c, 1m, 10m over a period of days or weeks, might be given to clear an aetiology such as vaccination or exposure to poisonous fumes or substances.

7. Prophylactic method

The first use of a homeopathic remedy in prophylaxis was done by Hahnemann, when he used the remedy belladonna as prophylaxis for scarlatina.

Boenninghausen successfully prevented smallpox with the use of variolinum, the nosode made from smallpox. Healthy people who took the remedy did not become infected with smallpox during an epidemic. Other examples include lathyrus sativa (a plant) for polio, pertussin (a preparation of the bacteria bordetella pertussis) for whooping cough, morbillinum for measles, diphtherinum for diphtheria.

Most of the experience with this approach was during the era preceding the availability of vaccines. Homeopaths reported a decrease in the severity and frequency of disease in those patients who received the nosode preventively.

The method of homeopathic prophylaxis has never been rigorously tested. Nonetheless, there is some evidence suggesting that homeopathic medicines do act to prevent diseases during epidemics.

With the increase in foreign travel from the early twentieth century onwards and the increased risk of exposure to tropical disease and foreign pathogens, homeopaths have prescribed nosodes in the same manner for travellers. More recently, with advent of vaccines and the increase in surgical and dentistry procedures, some homeopaths now prescribe a homeopathic prophylaxis before these events. This is believed to lessen the detrimental effects of these procedures on the body.

Appropriate times to use this method

- When there is a risk of exposure to a foreign pathogen, for example during an epidemic or when travelling.
- As a prophylaxis before a planned traumatic event such as vaccination, dentistry or surgery.

Prescription guidelines

Generally a single dose, split dose or a collective split dose of 30c or 200c is given in the event of exposure or prior to a trauma, although a prescription may be determined by the case.

8. Detox therapeutic method

when not used as part of the layers method

This method involves the removal of the residual toxins in the system which may be affecting the patient's state of health and/or causing new symptoms. The procedure is the same as that for the drug layer of the layers method but it is independent of the structure of the layers method. Therefore, it can be used at any stage in a patient's course of treatment, without presenting pathology.

Appropriate times to use this method

- In cases of long-term drug use unrelated to pathology such as vaccines, birth control pill, HRT and blood pressure tablets.
- In cases of recreational drug use or abuse without pathology.
- In chronic or acute cases.
- When there has been over-exposure to toxins in general.

Prescription guidelines

A detox therapeutic is reached by differentiating between remedies that have:

- a detoxifying action
- an affinity for the liver
- and are fitting to the case.

Detox therapeutics are given in a low potency, 6–30c or 6x–30x, with frequent repetition, up to four times daily. A tip to help find your main detox remedies quickly is look in a therapeutics book for the key remedies that have an affinity for the liver or kidneys for example cheladonium, berberis vulgaris and nux vomica.

Detoxifying patients

The detoxification of patients is often used as part of an overall treatment programme. There are many ways of approaching this. These are evolving and being developed by homeopaths using them in clinical practice.

Three approaches in common use are

- Organ support
- The Singh approach
- Bowel nosode programme

Organ support

This approach involves identifying weakened organs in the system and prescribing remedies that are known to have an affinity for those organs in order to bring about improved function.

Remedies are selected for their close affinity for the organ and similarity to the symptoms of weakness and dysfunction that are being presented.

If the organ in question is weakened through functional disturbance we call this prescription an **organ support therapeutic.**

If however, the organ has been compromised through pathology and/or prolonged drug use, then although the process is the same it is known as **organ drainage therapeutic**.

Sarcodes (remedies prepared from the tissue of a healthy organ) are prescribed as support remedies for weakened organs and, when given alongside other homeopathic remedies, are believed to act like a homing device, directing the action of the remedy to the specific organ in need.

Other approaches used for organ support are biochemic tissue salts (also known as Schüssler's tissue salts) and herbal tinctures. Herbal tinctures can also be used as an organ drainage therapeutic.

Appropriate times to use this approach

- If organs or systems need to be detoxified or strengthened before administering the indicated remedy. It is not appropriate to give organ remedies when there is no organ dysfunction, disease, or toxicity.
- Alongside other methods to strengthen the body's weakest parts.
- In pathology where there is prolonged drug use.
- To reduce aggravations.
- In cases where the patient is too weak or too sensitive to respond well to other forms of prescribing.
- In chronic cases.

Organ support is often used alongside other methods as a way of aiding the system in the process of healing. It is especially helpful during periods of detoxification, as aggravations are reduced while the body discharges.

Prescription guidelines

In general tinctures are used in their complete form to maintain their healing integrity and are rich in compounds that have beneficial effects on certain systems and organs to treat, cure or prevent disease. They can stimulate the immune system, stimulate the regeneration of a damaged liver to repair itself, or balance the endocrine system.

Prescribing organ therapeutics

There are two types of tinctures available:

Herbal tinctures are made up from various herbs using a dilution ratio of one part to three parts of alcohol (up to 35% proof). From a material perspective they are considered to be stronger than homeopathic mother tinctures as they contain more of the organic matter (and therefore essential nutrients and vitamins).

Homeopathic mother tinctures are also made from herbs and are used extensively by many homeopaths for organ support. The key difference between mother tinctures and herbal tinctures is their dilution rate and the strength of the alcohol used. Mother tinctures have an alcohol ratio of one part to nine parts alcohol (up to 95% proof) and so in theory although they are seen as weaker than herbal tinctures as they contain less of the original material they should also be seen as more potent in terms of alcohol content.

Some homeopaths find the **biochemic tissue salts** a useful addition to their tool-kit. They are made in the same way as homeopathic remedies in 3x, 6x or 9x potencies. According to Schüssler's theory, any disturbance in the molecular motion of one of the twelve cell salts in living tissues, caused by a deficiency in the requisite amount, constitutes disease which can be balanced and healed by prescribing the same mineral salts in small quantities. The action of biochemic tissue salts is at a very cellular level and they act as nourishment for the organ.

Low potency organ-specific remedies are made in the same way as other homeopathic remedies and are prescribed no higher than 6x with frequent repetition. Low potency remedies that have an organ affinity are best prepared in water and prescribed at five drops on the tongue, three times daily.

The Singh approach

This is based on the work of Pritam Singh and is a form of detox therapeutics. It is useful for patients whose symptoms are a result of toxicity in the body. It is used to remove 'obstacles to cure' which may be affecting the patient's state of health and/or causing symptoms. It is thought to be useful to:
- Remove residual toxins from different organ systems.
- Remove miasmatic blocks.

It can be used at any stage in a patient's course of treatment, even when there is no presenting pathology.
This approach can be used once you have a clear understanding of the general level of toxicity, weakened organ systems, the miasmatic blocks and likely obstacles to cure.
It was originally described in the book *Classical Homeopathy Revisited* by Roger Dyson and Jean Cole. It involves a regime of giving miasmatic nosodes including psorinum, tuberculinum, and medorrhinum in descending potencies along with organ support and drainage remedies.

Appropriate times to use this approach

- In cases of miasmatic blocks, organ dysfunction and obstacles to cure, such as long-term drug use unrelated to pathology, for example vaccines, birth control pill, HRT or blood pressure tablets.
- In cases of recreational and prescribed drug use or abuse without pathology.
- When there are obvious obstacles to cure such as an over-exposure to toxins in general.
- In chronic or acute cases.

Potency

This approach introduces the concept of descending potency in order to maximise the potential of the remedy. This is because aggravations are minimised and different patients respond individually to different potencies, and so by using the full range you are more likely to get a positive result with all cases!
The potencies used are 10M, 1M, 200c, 30c, 18c, 12c and 6c.

Occasionally the CM potency is used. Lower descending potencies are used if the patient has:

- a medical history of a serious nature that may be fatal
- is over 60 years
- poor vitality, poor recovery rate for acute and chronic conditions
- an irregular pulse, unless medical investigation have shown that there is no underlying problem.

Any aggravations with the high potencies can be curtailed by giving a lower potency

Prescription guidelines

This approach has evolved and changed so that most cases are now opened with rad-brom, berberis vulgaris and kali-phos. Rad-brom is used to break through blockages and enhance the action of remedies. Berberis is used after rad-brom for support for the excretory organs and kali-phos as support for the nervous system. The indicated remedy is then given followed by an indicated miasmatic remedy or obstacle to cure remedy.

Bowel nosode programme

Bowel cancer is now a major problem and leads to many deaths. Homeopaths have had to develop ways of dealing with patients with this and other diseases that appear to be linked to bowel problems. Historically homeopaths have used 'nosodes' which are homeopathic remedies prepared from actual disease tissue or a disease-associated organism. Dr Edward Bach introduced the idea of prepared remedies from non-lactose fermenting bacilli from the intestinal tract, hence the term 'bowel nosodes' (occasionally called the 'intestinal nosodes').

Twelve bowel nosodes were originally listed in Agrawal's *A Treatise on Bowel Nosodes*. More recently Doris Beauchamp has devised a treatment sequence based on eight of these (morgan pure; sycotic co; morgan gaertner; proteus; gaertner; dysentery co; bacillus no. 7; and bacillus no.10). Each has an association with specific polycrest remedies and tissue salts. Your selection is determined by the case. Doris uses this programme to support her normal prescribing methods.

Appropriate times to use this programme

- In chronic and acute cases.
- When the nosode is the indicated remedy based on the presenting symptom picture.
- When the indicated remedy fails to act or cure.
- When the symptom picture is unclear and too mixed-up to fathom.
- When the action of an indicated remedy does not hold and the state relapses.
- When acute states do not resolve with the indicated remedy and become sub-acute or chronic states – use as an intercurrent throughout layers prescribing.

Prescription guidelines

The bowel nosodes are prescribed at 200c single dose, followed 8 days later by an appropriate polycrest remedy at 10M and then tissue salts at 6x or 9x. 1,2,or 3 x daily for three weeks. This may be repeated every 5 – 6 weeks for about a year.

Summary

As a modern homeopath you need to have a clear understanding of the main methods to be able to treat the modern patient appropriately. The essence of becoming a successful homeopath is simply the art of applying different methods to suit the individual needs of your patient so that healing can be accomplished in the most speedy, gentle and reliable manner.

No approach is sufficient on its own and all methods have their limitations due to the time and context of when they were developed. However, by understanding the different methods you can begin to be creative and this ensures that homeopathy continues to grow, develop and evolve to meet the ever-increasing levels of suppression and toxicity that our twenty-first century patients will present.

You should understand clearly

- exactly what method you are using
- where you are aiming your prescription
- what you expect that prescription to do
- where you will go next if the prescription doesn't work.

It saddens me to hear homeopaths blaming remedies for aggravations or being afraid of remedies. The remedies are not the problem. The issue is how you are prescribing them and your inability to listen to the vital energy of the patient when it tells you quite clearly you are prescribing in the wrong place because you are using the wrong method of applying homeopathy. Homeopathy is a really safe system of medicine. It is a very different paradigm from the concepts underlying allopathy because one is an energy medicine that supports the body to heal itself, while the other is preoccupied with eliminating and suppressing symptoms without understanding the impact of such an action on the patient.

There is no one method that is perfect nor is there one method that defines homeopathy as a system of medicine.

What defines homeopathy

- our ability to understand the causes of disturbances in the vital energy of our patients
- our ability to find remedies that stimulate the process of self-healing
- the way we make our energy remedies.

Classical homeopathy, which is a single method approach, has its place and context for use, just as a tautopathic approach has its appropriate use in practice. If you are taught to look at patients from one perspective with only one tool in your tool-kit the results will be limited. The endless arguments about what method a practitioner uses are pointless because the methods of application are not homeopathy, merely tools that help us to achieve our common aim – that of healing. The question you should be asking is how good are the tools I'm using? And am I getting the results my patients are expecting from me? If you aren't, then it is time to look at new methods of application and not frantically hunt for new and obscure remedies to rescue you, the patient or homeopathy.

You should now have an overview of

- the concept of part-patient methods
- the eight recognised part-patient methods
- having a good working knowledge of the principles behind each method
- some homeopathic approaches to detoxification programmes for patients
- the art of applying different methods to suit the individual needs of your patient
- how to research each method further.

In the next chapter we review the difference between methods, diagnostic tools and ethics in an effort to clarify some of the reasons why homeopathy appears such a divided profession. Methods are part of the 'tools' of homeopathy not homeopathy itself and I suggest that it is the misunderstanding of these terms which leads to so much division and angst among homeopaths.

Very few of us can think clearly about the habitual way we think, about the 'mindset' out of which we judge the 'rightness' and 'value' of everything

Robert Davidson

Chapter 6

Methods, ethics, diagnostic tools and practical homeopathy

We have defined the meaning of a method as 'the mode or rule used in carrying out a task or accomplishing an aim; an orderly procedure'.

Methods are the different ways of applying homeopathy that have developed over the past 200 years. They are really ways of approaching the same problem – that of how to most effectively and efficiently prescribe the most appropriate remedies for the individual patient. In essence the different methods use different styles and place a slightly different emphasis on the varying factors that are important when prescribing homeopathically.

Don't confuse 'methods' with ethics

The word 'ethics', derived from old French 'ethiques' and Greek 'ethika', refers to a system of moral principles governing the appropriate conduct for a person or group. Medical ethics is the discipline of evaluating the merits, risks and social concerns of activities in the field of medicine. Every major medical organisation in the world supports a set of 'ethical practices' or a 'code of conduct' which regulate the physicians associated with that particular organisation. These codes lay down a certain set of standards for professional conduct by the physicians, keeping in mind the best interests of the patients.

As professional bodies, many homeopathic organisations have a code of conduct and a set of ethical practices for their members. While the basis remains the same, there are some differences in these codes. The reason for this is the lack of uniform regulation and laws which regulate homeopathic practice in various countries. While in some countries, such as India, homeopathy is well recognised and there are definite laws governing its practice, in most western countries there are no separate laws which deal with homeopathy – although this is slowly changing. In some places you need to be a conventional medical doctor to practice homeopathy and in others you don't need any qualification at all. The education structure also varies from country to country.

Uniform standards of practice are difficult to achieve as long as there is such disparity in the state and the status of homeopathy in different countries. However we should question the need for such uniformity as it may not necessarily be conducive to the healing of the patient as one of the principles of homeopathy is individualisation of treatment!

It is important not to confuse 'standards for professional conduct' for homeopaths with the different methods that are tools of the trade or with 'the principles of homeopathy'. Much of the divisiveness is caused by people confusing these three areas and trying to make their opinion the deciding factor.

Homeopathy is a science. Samuel Hahnemann attempted to develop homeopathic practice for over 50 years. He produced a set of principles that have laid the basis of the science of homeopathy for the past 200 years. However, as with most 'founding fathers' of any discipline, his followers and his critics have continued to build on, develop and change his original concept and this has led to much controversy as to what true homeopathy is.

Within homeopathy, as within any profession and scientific discipline there are many factions – single remedy prescribers, multiple remedy prescribers, combination prescribers, people who prescribe solely on mental symptoms or pathology and many others. The different types of prescription depend on exactly what you are trying to cure and the different methods act as a guide to help practitioners get clear about what they are doing. There is nothing wrong with diversity within the profession as long as practitioners do not get muddled about what they are trying to do. You can use any 'method' as long as it is based on the principles of homeopathy and you act within the standards of professional conduct.

Unfortunately there is a tendency for people to adopt a very dogmatic and religious approach to homeopathy and for each faction to call its 'method' right (and therefore see the others as wrong!).

Many people feel that there has never been any consensus on 'what is homeopathy' but I feel that this is not so. The fundamentals were laid down by Hahnemann and have been consistently proved and adapted by many eminent homeopaths since, in the same way as any scientific discipline. The methods presented in this book all follow the basic principles. None of them are right or wrong but you do need to know how to use them appropriately to achieve maximum healing potential for the patient. The underlying principles don't change.

Some believe that in recent years the situation has only worsened with more homeopaths coming up with more 'schools of thought' and more divisiveness within the community – not just on principles but also on gurus that people follow! My understanding of this phenomenon of 'guru worship' is that it fits well with guestamology and remedy chasing. It will attract those homeopaths who, lacking confidence in both homeopathy and their own ability to practice it are, in essence, seeking a saviour.

The proliferation of 'schools of thought' can also be seen from a positive perspective as homeopaths continually develop their knowledge and gain a deeper understanding of how homeopathy works. They are also trying to find more effective ways of getting results for their patients while at the same time the patients are presenting more complex cases.

There should be no confusion as to 'what homeopathy is,' if the first seven principles are understood and the guiding principles of the law of cure and concepts of susceptibility are used as a base. The rest of the so called 'laws of homeopathy' are then used as reference tools, tested by empirical practice.

Methods and diagnostic tools

There are a number of other approaches to choosing remedies that are currently taught and used by practitioners. I have not addressed them in this book because I feel they are not sufficiently developed within an empirical scientific framework, for example dream provings, meditation provings, and psychic approaches (pendulum, tarot etc).

Neither have I included iridology, kinesiology, facial diagnosis and the use of radionics and bio-resonance machines as these are diagnostic tools and not methods. I will now address these briefly and attempt to place them in a context that will enable you to understand how they are used by some homeopaths.

Diagnostic tools

Homeopathy is a non-invasive medical practice and most homeopaths are not trained to carry out medical examinations unless they are already nurses or doctors. However even a homeopath needs to be trained to use some basic medical instruments to examine their patients. The most-used ones in clinics are:

- blood pressure monitor
- tongue depressor
- torch
- stethoscope
- otoscope (for ears).

These are physical tools to help you do your job in the same way as a carpenter needs a saw.

The next level of tools available to you are those that are essentially aids to observation and diagnosis. In this category come the following:

Facial and tongue analysis: facial analysis has been part of Chinese medicine for thousands of years and is a fairly well developed and recorded diagnostic tool. It can be used as a simple observational tool by almost everyone, but can also be studied and developed to a very high level under the right teacher. The tongue is seen as a key part of facial diagnosis as it is called the 'mirror of the stomach'. It is a highly active, sensitive organ, which is the beginning and the only visible part of the digestive tract. It can help you to determine many conditions and the overall health of the body. The healthy tongue is free of any discomfort, such as pain, stinging, burning, swelling, excrescences or numbness. It is moist, with a rough surface, and has an evenly coloured pink surface overlaying pale red. Inspection of the patient's tongue is, therefore, a very useful starting point in most consultations and can be cross-referenced using a repertory.

Eye analysis and iridology: most health practitioners will have observed that the eyes are the 'mirror of the soul' and can give a lot of information about the state of health of the patient. The eyes have a long history as a diagnostic tool and they also feature in practices such as NLP (neuro linguistic programming) as an aid to communication skills. Iridology is a fairly advanced diagnostic tool and is often studied either with homeopathy or as an additional diagnostic skill for practitioners.

Fingernail analysis: the appearance and colour of our nails not only reflects the status of our health but can give valuable information about the underlying disease condition. Having an insight into the varying states of fingernails and their underlying pathology can help us to select the most appropriate remedy.

We now move on to another level of diagnosis which is based on using approaches to health developed more recently. These often claim to be health disciplines in their own right but do not have the long history of empirical research that homeopathy has.

Kinesiology: a natural health care system which uses gentle muscle testing to evaluate many functions of the body in the structural, chemical, neurological and biochemical realms. Kinesiology testing does not diagnose disease. Muscle testing enables analysis which detects minor functional imbalances. Minor imbalances, when not corrected, accumulate and cause compensations. Compensations compound each other, lead to functional changes, and give rise to symptoms of discomfort, pain or maybe allergic reactions. If these warnings are ignored, disease can follow. Kinesiology is essentially a body therapy which uses touch and massage to help patients deal with structural imbalances and energy blocks. It also often covers nutrition and supplements for nutritional deficiencies as part of the treatment. Kinesiology balances the whole person, enhancing health and well-being and thus warding off disease. It is seen as a preventive health intervention. Many homeopaths are now adding a knowledge of kinesiology to their tool-kit to help support their practice.

Radionics and bio-resonance machines: this is a new and developing field based on devices using harmonic frequencies which have a positive influence on human regulatory mechanism. The oldest kind of biological resonance is sunlight. If light, as the electro-magnetic oscillation of a defined frequency, touches our skin, it triggers off other energetic processes such as pigmentation or the formation of vitamin D. It is obvious that a large number of other frequencies, besides that of ultra-violet light, also have some kind of effect on the organism. In the medical field, biological resonance means seeking the frequencies necessary for the stimulation and final regulation of the organism. Increasingly homeopaths are now using bio-resonance machines as diagnostic tools and this is a rapidly developing market. (A word of warning – if you do not understand the principles of homeopathy and how to use different methods appropriately these machines just become a technical version of guestamology leading to further remedy chasing!)

Naturopathy: the practice of naturopathy is the provision of guidance, specialist advice and the use of natural therapeutics to help the person achieve optimum health and prevent disease. The practicing naturopath uses skills and experience which are broadly based and include, among others, homeopathy, herbal medicine, nutritional medicine and acupuncture. The naturopath, in selecting the most appropriate form of therapy, will use established diagnostic procedures such as kinesiology, bio-resonance, case-taking, dowsing or electro-acupuncture. Naturopathy is very much in tune with the underlying principles of homeopathy and many homeopaths are seeing it as a natural post-graduate progression and in line with a continuing professional development approach.

Nutrition: is one of the most important aspects of health. (We are what we eat!) Many studies have been done on the link between poor nutrition and disease, especially on the long-term effects of a refined carbohydrate diet. In the West, diets are not particularly healthy due to a high intake of refined carbohydrates, irregular eating habits and the use of stimulants such as alcohol, nicotine, caffeine and recreational drugs, leading to deficiency in nutrition. The vast majority of patients will be coming to see you in this state of malnutrition. Without the basic building blocks to heal tissue some patients may not respond well to homeopathic remedies. The ability to recognise nutritional deficiencies and know how to support patients where necessary has always been part of the homeopathic approach and is becoming even more important today.

'Practical' homeopathy and methods

I feel at this point it is important to explain the ethos of *practical* homeopathy and to define it with clarity for readers who are confused about the name and what this means in relationship to the study of different methods of homeopathy.

Most importantly practical homeopathy is not and has never been intended to be a *method*.

Practical homeopathy is an approach to the study and practice of homeopathy that is based on the principles of homeopathy. We encourage students to apply those principles in real life and to learn from the successes and failures of their own and others' experience, both as homeopaths and as practitioners in the 'business' of homeopathy. One common misunderstanding is caused by people who say they teach 'classical' and 'practical' homeopathy. This implies that 'practical' homeopathy is a method which it is not!

Practical homeopathy teaches a range of 'methods' that have been developed since Hahnemann's time. A training based on practical homeopathy requires you to understand what needs to be cured, if there are any obstacles to cure, how to choose an appropriate method, and to understand why a particular method is suitable for the individual. It provides you with a range of tools and concepts that increases your ability to treat patients successfully.

Why is the practical approach becoming more popular?

All disciplines grow and develop on the work done by those that preceded them and homeopathy is no exception to this. We have discussed the stages of prescribing in Chapter 1 – the primitive, sophisticated, degenerative and current 'collapse' stage where large numbers of the population begin to suffer from a total immune system breakdown such as AIDS, allergies and all kinds of cancers.

Dealing with this level of toxicity and its effects has become a major part of practice, and the successful practitioner will need strategies for dealing with this.

The implication of this for the homeopath is that methods for prescribing are no longer as clear cut. The complex pictures presented by the modern patient need to be matched by an understanding of the variety of methods that are available, and which particular method is the most appropriate at particular points along the healing process. Hence the development of practical homeopathy.

What has been found in practice is that for homeopathy to be effective and simple it requires different methods of applying the basic homeopathic principles. One method may work well in one situation but can be difficult to apply in another. A 'practically' trained homeopath may well decide to use the classical method if it is considered the most appropriate for their patient. So classical homeopathy, which is a single method approach, has its place and context for use, just a detox therapeutic approach has its appropriate use in practice. If you are taught to look at patients from only one perspective with only one tool in your tool-kit the results are limited.

A practical homeopath therefore is someone who has been trained to be able to use a number of different ways to approach a patient's case. These are called methods.

Practical homeopaths 'stand where they can see the view', focus on the present and do not rely exclusively on methods that worked well for nineteenth and twentieth century patients. We look at where we are now and are open to continually adopting new proven methods for the future in order to keep making homeopathy work. Hahnemann was the first practical homeopath in the sense that he never stopped changing and adapting his approach.

In the next chapter I give a personal perspective on the role methods have played in my own development as a successful homeopath. I also discuss some of the issues and criticisms that arise among homeopaths once you begin to cover a range of methods both in teaching and in practice.

Minds are like parachutes...they work best when open

Lord Thomas Dewar

Chapter 7

A personal perspective

Over the past few years I have had the privilege of working with many homeopaths – students, new graduates and experienced professionals from a range of colleges and backgrounds across the country. I am increasingly finding many graduates leaving college with an underlying sense of fear about homeopathy and with a limited understanding of methods. If these have been covered at all then they are often taught from theory only and in a confused way. Theoretically they have this wonderful list of tools but in practical terms little idea of how to apply them properly.

This style of education appears to be producing homeopaths who are at best excellent totality prescribers, and at worst, refined in the art of guestamology.

There is much confusion about the basic principles and methods, adherence to all kinds of homeopathic myths and I feel this leads to 'guru worship' and remedy chasing, attracting those homeopaths who lack confidence in both homeopathy and their own ability to practice it.

Over the years, as my own practice developed, I began to learn about the art of homeopathy, the vital energy of each of my patients and what worked in practice. I realised that what worked was having a thorough understanding of what was going on with each patient and developing a strategy that suited each person. I see this now as exercising due diligence on a case, understanding causations and applying the method of prescribing appropriately, as Robin Murphy used to say 'aetiology over symptomology'. What I was never taught, nor could I find out from any book or tutor, was the context for choosing the method or for the symptoms. Finding the right context for choosing a method is very important because this allows you to individualise your case.

As this realisation struck, I began my true journey as a homeopath, supported by the faith many of my patients had in my abilities to help them. I know homeopathy works, and it is easy to make it work if you understand what is going on with your patient. Homeopathy is a gentle, easy and effective system of medicine but most of us are taught it back to front by focusing on the remedy, and not on the people we are supposed to be curing. Using a time-line to help understand the context of the disease is a valuable tool because the answer to your patient's problems is in their case. Learn to be a good detective because if you cannot make your way back to the cause you will never get a cure and at best you will merely palliate the symptoms.

Hahnemann's guiding principles are of great value to the intrepid homeopath seeking to gain maximum results for their patient. They are:

'Every homeopath must have a good understanding of what causes and sustains illness and how to eliminate it from healthy people.

'To cure a patient, the homeopath must discover the occurrence of the exciting, underlying cause through understanding the individuality of the patient, their constitution (mental, emotions, physicals etc).

'The unprejudiced observer must be fully aware of the central state through perceptible signs. In every individual case of disease, the totality of the symptoms must be the homeopath's principle concern.'

These guiding principles brought me right back to the importance of understanding the context of my patient's disease. When Hahnemann talks of the totality of the symptoms it is within the context of disease – understanding what needs to be cured and what is the best method for achieving that cure.

To help me find the right context for my patient's symptoms, I borrowed the idea of developing a time-line as a case management tool from Dr Eizayaga and Dr Elmiger. The development of a time-line allows you to step back and overview your case, it makes you the 'unprejudiced observer' and gives you the context of where your patient's symptoms have come from; this will lead to a method that is the most appropriate for your patient at this point. Symptoms come from somewhere, you need to find out where they come from and once you understand that the method falls into place. The context of the patient's symptoms should guide you to the method.

It is important to understand that the methods of prescribing were developed by many different homeopaths over time and that I am not claiming authorship of any particular method or promoting one method as 'the way' to practice. Nor am I putting the methods in a hierarchy of importance or, even worse, denigrating certain methods as not being 'homeopathy'.

Methods are tools that should be used appropriately. They are not set in stone as 'rules and regulations'. We can't use nineteenth century methods for twenty-first century patients (in this respect 'totality mentality prescribing' will leave you frustrated and demoralised if it is the only tool you have!)

As Hahnemann said 'The homeopath must be attentive and faithfully record the individual nature of the case'. An understanding of subtle energy can help you do this. Once you master the art of applying different methods to different cases you will begin to create your own successful practice.

Isn't having different methods confusing?

It's only confusing if you have not been taught properly how to apply them to meet the needs of individual patients. Particularly in your early years of practice, the advantage of having different methods is that it gives a flexibility and range of clinical choices which can only be appreciated by those who know how to use them for the benefit of patients.

Do not listen to those who have not seriously used the various methods but question their value. That is like asking an allopath about homeopathy. Confusion is a natural state for those homeopaths who have not been taught to apply different methods appropriately and is what they get used to. (It is how you may feel most of the time with patients, but it does not help to suppress confusion with false certainty and a dogmatic belief that the one method you know is the only way of applying homeopathy).

It is important that you understand the process of working with methods and then use them, experiment with them appropriately and continue to learn from your experience. This will help both the student and practitioner to work within the natural confusion of practice and find the appropriate method for each unique patient.

Is homeopathy dangerous?

No it is not dangerous – the fact that after 200 years it is still available as an over the counter medicine in most countries should speak for itself. I have never seen homeopathy harm, kill, mutilate, cripple or injure anyone. If it were possible to kill sick people easily then students would do it in large numbers, as trainee allopaths do. I have seen no evidence of this in **The College of Practical Homeopathy** student clinic.

It is true that some patients are very fragile, often from allopathic poisoning, surgery or radiation and chemical poisoning. It is important to recognise the fragile patient. The evidence of the importance of applying different methods appropriately can be seen in student clinics where complex cases with multiple levels of poisoning and allopathic intervention have been skillfully treated. If students can do it, so can you. Homeopathy is always safe. If anyone tells you differently then it is because they have misunderstood what they are supposed to be doing as homeopaths. And even then they could not claim to have killed anyone. Having a choice of methods means that the homeopath can, with knowledge and simple insight use the method best suited to the patient whether that patient be weak or strong. This makes for consistent good results.

Finally...

A great homeopath once said to me 'there is no room for fear in homeopathy' and through my journey to becoming a homeopath I began to understand what he meant.

Fear is quite normal when you are confused about your tools or what it is you are supposed to be curing. If you feel fearful it is because you are not clear what you are doing. Sometimes when you go down the wrong path, and remedies do not work, you need to backtrack to get on firm ground. A good approach for this is to review the time-line and the reasons behind your choice of method to see if another method would suit better. Or you could start again at this point – choosing a method which suits the patient's case *at this point* (as you would do if you were taking over a case from another homeopath). Don't let fear kill your creativity or prevent you from exploring new methods of applying homeopathy. There are many different simple ways of curing the sick – a choice of methods enhances the flexibility and creativity of the true healer and allows the simple power of homeopathy to help you. That is real healing.

'Homeopathy is life's best chance to heal itself'. If you find yourself being frightened or intimidated by anyone in homeopathy then you should avoid him or her like the plague – for suppressed fear in many disguises is indeed contagious and will affect the whole of your career as a homeopath.

You, the reader, can make up your own minds but in my experience homeopathy is truly the most exciting and enjoyable way of living for anyone who wants to heal sick people. You should not let those who would limit homeopathy to what they do and nothing else intimidate you or otherwise limit the possibility of an exciting and enjoyable future as a student or practitioner.

I hope you have both enjoyed and been challenged by this book, and that it has gone some way to filling any gaps in your understanding of the range and use of the different methods available within the field of homeopathy.

Bibliography & reference books

Homeopathy Revisited	Rudolph Verspoor & Patricia Lynn Smith
A Guide to Methodologies of Homeopathy ISBN 0951765701	Ian Watson
Indications of Miasm (Indian Edition)	Choudhry
Classical Homeopathy Revisited ISBN 1-874581-04-5	Jean Cole & Roger Dyson
Treatise on Homoeopathic Medicine	Francisco Eizayaga
Rediscovering Real Medicine ISBN: 1 84333 190	Dr.J Elmiger
Miasmatic Prescribing ISBN: 0 95421 124 0 1	Dr. S. Banerjea
Homoeopathic Remedy Guide ISBN: 0 9635764	Robin Murphy
Homoeopathy in Epidemic Diseases ISBN: 0-85207-305-4	D.Shepherd
Treatise on the Bowel Nosodes	Dr.Y. Agrawal
Twelve tissue salts of Schüssler (Indian Edition)	Boericke & Dewey
Miracles of Healing (Indian Edition)	J Ellis Barker
New Lives for Old (Indian Edition)	J Ellis Barker
A Concise repertory of Homoeopathic Medicines (Indian Edition)	Dr S R Phatak